STRONG LIKE HER

STRONG LIKE HER

A CELEBRATION OF RULE BREAKERS, HISTORY MAKERS, AND UNSTOPPABLE ATHLETES

HALEY SHAPLEY

PHOTOGRAPHS BY SOPHY HOLLAND

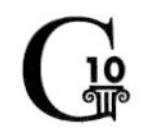

GALLERY BOOKS
New York London Toronto Sydney New Delhi

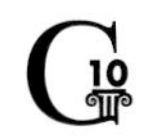

Gallery Books
An Imprint of Simon & Schuster, Inc.
1230 Avenue of the Americas
New York, NY 10020

First Gallery Books hardcover edition April 2020

Manufactured in the United States of America

10 9 8 7 6 5 4 3 2 1

Library of Congress Cataloging-in-Publication Data has been applied for.

ISBN 978-1-9821-2085-6
ISBN 978-1-9821-2087-0 (ebook)

To strong women everywhere

"You've always had the power."

—GLINDA THE GOOD WITCH

CONTENTS

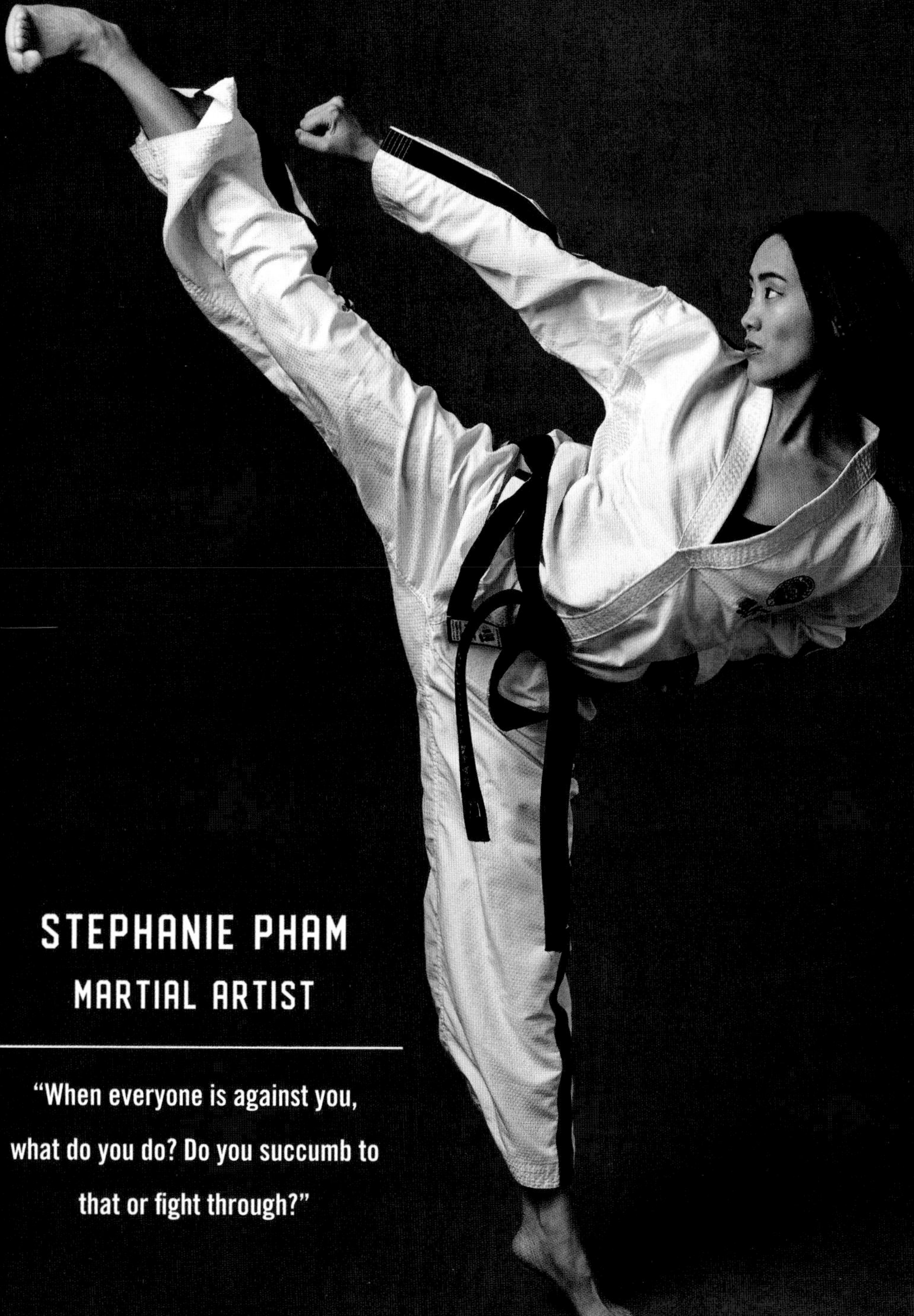

STEPHANIE PHAM

MARTIAL ARTIST

"When everyone is against you, what do you do? Do you succumb to that or fight through?"

INTRODUCTION

A few years ago, I decided to compete in a bodybuilding show. My goal was not to become a professional but to challenge myself in something new. I trained for the physical aspects, yes—seeing how I could transform my body with consistent effort fascinated me. But I took it up for the mental challenge, too. I'm happiest when I'm learning new things and seeing how far I can push the boundaries of my mind—which in bodybuilding also happens to be inextricably linked to the body, given that you have to stay incredibly focused to get through all the workouts, strict meal timings, and unending gallons of water. Even mindfulness comes into play when you're lifting, to make sure you're engaging the muscles you're intending to target.

I learned a lot through the experience, about discipline, consistency, and what one ounce of almonds looks like. I also learned that even today, people have certain ideas about how women should look, and when you step outside those bounds—particularly on purpose—it invites commentary.

It surprised me, although maybe it shouldn't have. I'd started lifting heavy weights about two years before, and I distinctly remember walking into my gym the first day and seeing a woman with broad shoulders. She was very strong and very nice, and I was very sure I never wanted to look like her. It wasn't until I realized how powerful I felt slinging around a barbell that I began to let go of my preconceived ideas about my body's appearance.

• • •

IT CAN TAKE TIME TO deprogram a lifetime's worth of messaging. I was born when Jane Fonda's workout videos were booming in popularity. Spandex and step aerobics reigned, and in the era following Title IX, a civil rights law that banned discrimination in educational programs, girls were encouraged to play sports—or at least not overtly discouraged from it. I tried my hand (and feet) at lots of different things—ballet, gymnastics, soccer, track, swimming—before settling into basketball as my main sport. I spent hours at practice, and in that time, I worked to be more agile, smarter, more flexible, faster, more coordinated, and even smaller. Aside from some fleeting frustration in elementary school when I couldn't do a pull-up, I didn't spend much time thinking about strength. It never really occurred to me to be stronger.

To be fair, strength was not a common goal for girls when I was young. A 1985 quote from film critic Roger Ebert articulates the bias that I had probably internalized. "At first sight, there is something disturbing about a woman with massive muscles," he wrote in reference to *Pumping Iron II*, a movie about women's bodybuilding. "She is not merely androgynous, a combination of the sexes like an Audrey Hepburn or a Mick Jagger, but more like a man with a woman's face. We are so trained to equate muscles with men, softness and a slight build with women, that it seems nature has made a mistake."

Since then, the world has changed, and I have changed along with it. My weight today would horrify my eighteen-year-old self, and my arms are no longer the toothpicks I once prized. And yet I've learned the numbers on the scale are just one aspect of my life. It turns out I'm more motivated by the number I can deadlift.

Discovering the benefits of throwing around weights much heftier than eight-pound dumbbells has been life-changing, and I'm certainly not the only one to feel this way. Scroll through social media or peek inside a gym, and you're bound to spot women who are getting strong and loving it.

"I thought lifting was so cool from the first time I saw it," says professional strongwoman competitor Kristin Rhodes. "I was born to pick up anything heavy."

I was born to pick up anything heavy. When in history is that a sentence that could have been reasonably uttered by a woman? Maybe Katie Sandwina said it. She was a beloved circus performer who could lift a 600-pound cannon and bend iron bars. Or perhaps Pudgy Stockton said it. The "Queen of Muscle Beach" dazzled crowds in the 1940s by holding her husband in a handstand over her head, a feat she performed with curled hair and the curves that were popular in her day (yet make no mistake, Pudgy was jacked).

Stockton and others paved the way for the likes of Jan Todd, who set more than sixty national and world records in powerlifting; for Misty Copeland, whose muscular frame broke the mold of what a ballerina looks like; and even for me, a writer and first-time bodybuilding competitor who will never be famous for anything related to athletics.

AS I STARTED ON MY own strength journey, I began to think about where my aversion to visible muscularity had come from. Even though I'd played plenty of sports, when I walked into a weight room, I initially underestimated what I was capable of. Why was that? When my strength training came up, why did people warn me about how I was bound to hurt myself instead of encouraging me to test my limits? And why was I suddenly getting so many comments wondering whether I was worried about how I was appearing to the opposite sex, as if that had anything to do with my new hobby at all? I was seeing all kinds of strength being modeled by women in the public eye, and yet the topic was still so divisive.

I turned to one of my favorite places, the library, to answer some of these questions. But when I tried to read more about women and strength training throughout history, I came up mostly empty. Women were mentioned here and there, but the pages were dominated by men. I knew that couldn't be the whole story.

“I TRY TO NEVER FORGET THAT THE REASON I’M IN THE GYM IS BECAUSE I LOVE MY BODY AND I WANT IT TO BE STRONG.”

MEG GALLAGHER
POWERLIFTER

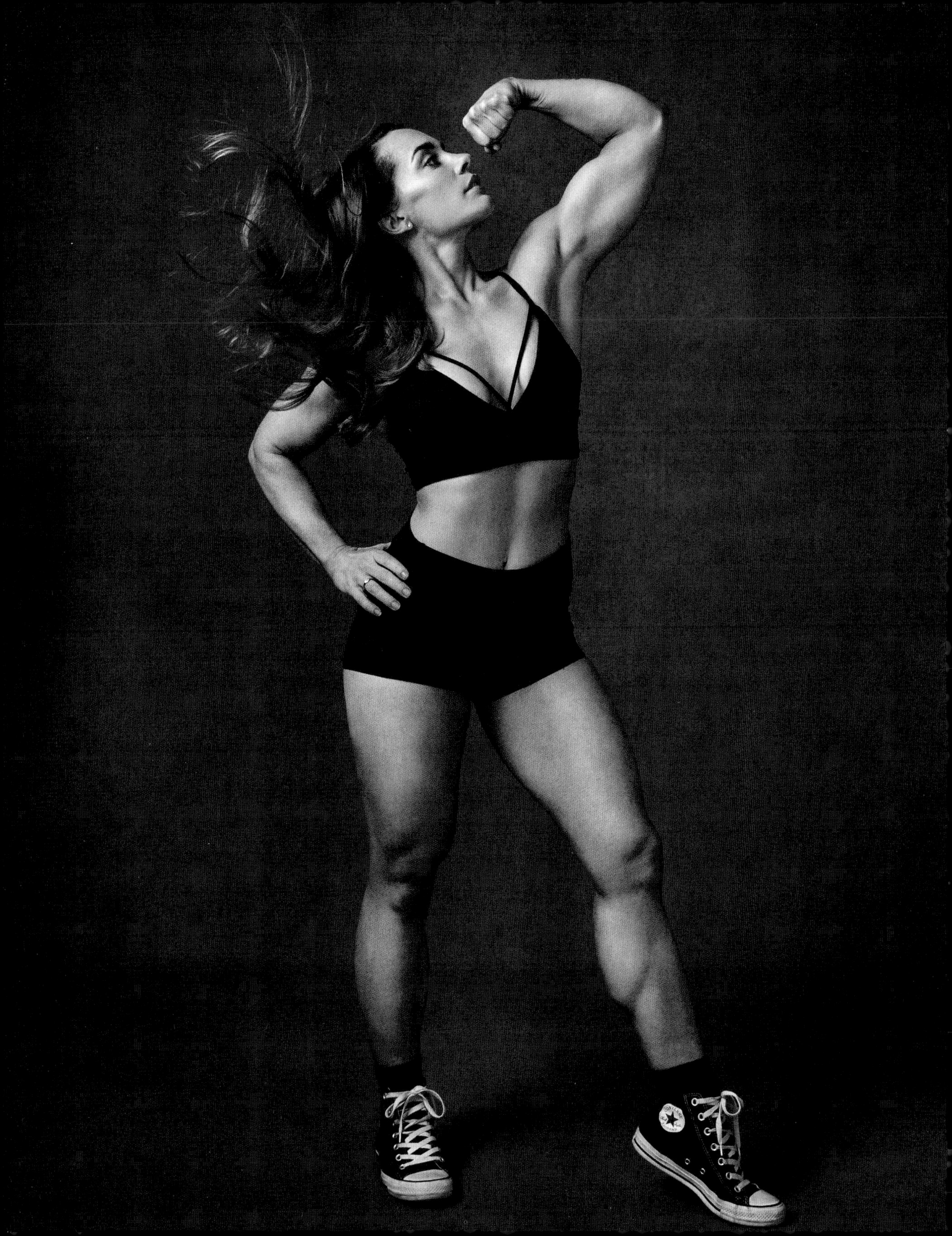

And so I set out to write about the women I knew had been kicking butt since the beginning of time, grappling with the issues surrounding strength long before I ever learned to front squat. What I didn't know was just how profound their contributions had been in ways that go beyond sports record books.

Throughout these chapters, we'll explore where our ideas about how women should look and act originate, uncovering biases that might feel hardwired but have actually been learned. We'll see how femininity and frailty once went hand in hand at the same time masculinity and muscularity came to be associated. We'll learn how women worked within the confines of social norms to stealthily get strong, eventually breaking down barriers even as they were governed by them. We'll dig into the cultural factors that have both encouraged and left some hesitant to build muscle, along with how strength served to expand a woman's role at key points in history. Mostly, we'll celebrate the awe-inspiring women, from ancient times to today, who have harnessed their physical power to great effect—which almost invariably serves to unlock strength in other areas of their lives.

This aspect has led to personal growth and social reform in ways that often go underrecognized. Physically strong women have been on the forefront of issues from suffrage to body autonomy to equality in the workplace. Knowing the history of women's hard-won freedoms is not only inspirational, it's instructive.

AS I COLLECTED THE STORIES of women through history who broke barriers and embraced strength despite convention, I found myself spotting their spiritual descendants everywhere I looked. In particular, I was struck by how female athletes of today continue to push the boundaries of what women are told they can (or cannot) do. The twenty-three contemporary female athletes profiled in this book model a new kind of female beauty, one based firmly in their incredible capacity and efforts. It seemed only right to include their photographs and their stories here. Their expertise ranges across disciplines, from rock climbing to martial arts to fencing. All exhibit strength in their own ways, adding to the definition of who and what a woman can be, and I'm personally inspired by each one. Without the women who were willing to swing a kettlebell before it was socially acceptable or learn to ride a bike in a corset and a full-length dress, we wouldn't be where we are today, in an age where strength sports are growing at a record pace. We have more to learn from these pioneers than *how* to get strong; *why* it's a worthy pursuit is the more powerful message.

As a woman's belief in her physical prowess grows, it does more than improve how much she can achieve athletically—it also elevates her overall well-being, including emotional, social, and economic health, and these are all signs of strength to strive for. No longer is her body an object to be judged; it's a vessel to be cultivated, and celebrated.

The warriors who rode on horseback in pants before that was "allowed," the swimmers who shed the weight of giant wool skirts to feel the freedom of cutting through the water, the runners who were told they could never have kids because their uteruses would fall out, the lifters who made do with equipment that wasn't designed for their proportions, and your neighbor who joined a boxing gym all share something special: the power of strength.

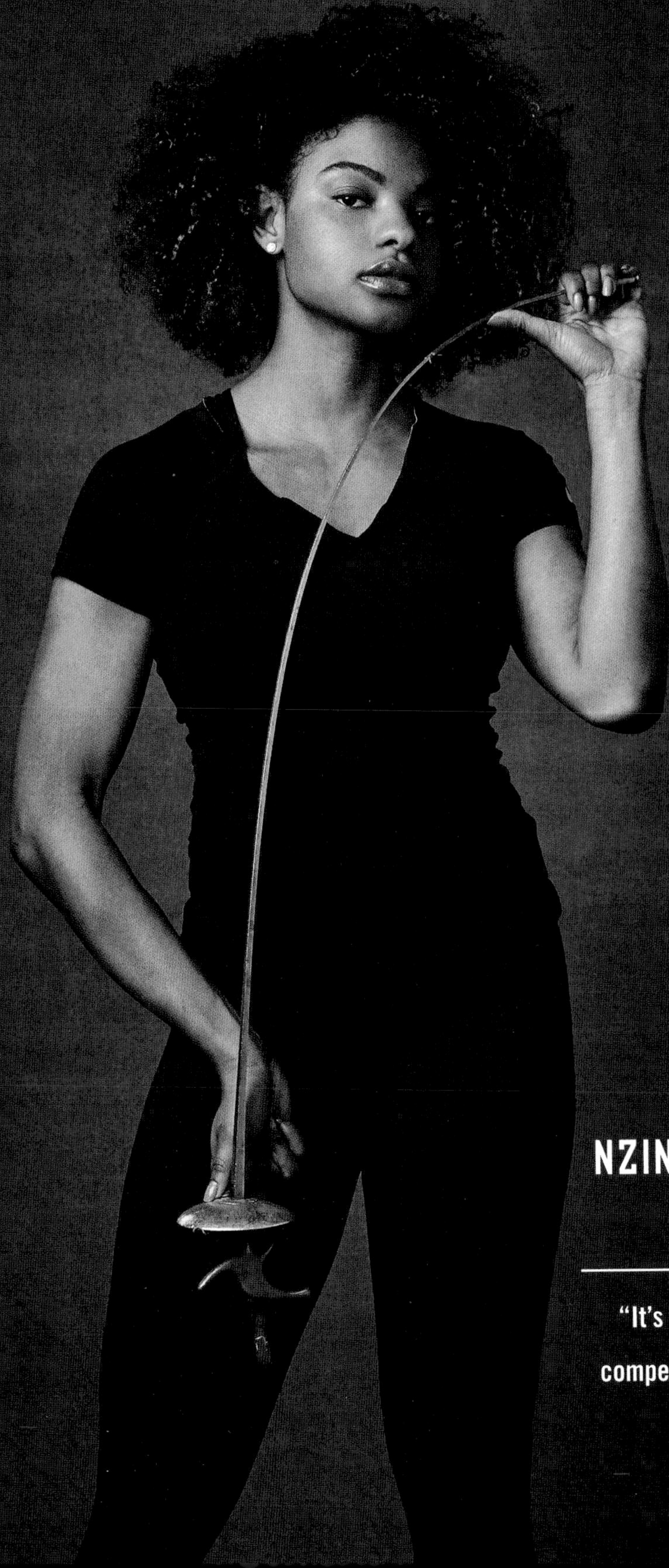

NZINGHA PRESCOD

FENCER

"It's always a goal when I'm competing to find my courage."

CHAPTER 1

THE ORIGINAL WARRIORS:
ANCIENT DEPICTIONS OF STRENGTH

The world's most famous athletic competition, the Olympic Games, began in 776 BCE in southern Greece. At the time, a law stipulated that if a married woman was found at the Olympic festival, she was to be thrown from Mount Typaeum into the river below. (Whether unmarried women were allowed to attend is unclear, but even if they were, it's probably not a stretch to say they weren't warmly welcomed.) To send a lady sailing over a cliff because she's curious seems a little harsh, especially for a culture that was so oriented on mind-body-spirit.

It's somewhat confusing as well, given what we know about how much the Greeks valued the gymnasium. Like contemporary gyms, the ancient Greek gymnasium was a place where one would train for physical competitions, as you might expect from the name, but it was also where young Greeks got their education in morals and ethics. The gymnasium was considered a central point of social and spiritual life, with athletics, academics, health, and well-being all intertwined. Throwing a javelin was just as important as discussing music theory.

But while the Greeks loved both sports and academia, there's a big asterisk next to that for the majority of the city-states: girls were not allowed to partake. Having a lively conversation about Pythagoras after wrestling practice was simply not a viable option for the average woman.

• • •

WHILE PHYSICAL EDUCATION FOR GIRLS was nowhere near on par with the boys, there were some opportunities to compete. Starting in the sixth century BCE, the Heraean Games offered a footrace for young, unmarried women. The distance was shorter than what the men ran on the same track, and instead of being nude, as the males were when running, the participants were covered in a one-shouldered tunic that hit just above the knee.

Something is better than nothing, but it wasn't nearly as prestigious as the Olympics, which remained resolutely male-only. The expectations were lower, as evidenced by the shorter distance, and the importance was lesser. Lots of rich detail about the Olympic Games has been passed through the generations, while the Heraean Games are far more mysterious. History was written by men, and men, by and large, wrote about themselves.

At least one woman tried to buck the system. In the fifth century BCE, Callipateira, mother of boxer Peisirodus, disguised herself as a male trainer in order to get into the Games. She had coached her son, after all, following the death of her husband, and she was just as knowledgeable about boxing as anyone else in the arena. When he won, she jumped over the fence to run to him, but unfortunately, her clothes got caught, and she was exposed—in more ways than one. In a show of mercy, organizers refrained from dumping her into the river, not on the basis that she had a rightful claim to attend but out of respect for her father, brothers, and son, who were all Olympic champions. Her own merits should have saved her, but instead, it was the men in her life. In the aftermath, a law was passed that trainers had to enter the Games naked, to double-check that they had the right parts to be there.

Callipateira wasn't the only Greek woman with a rebellious streak. The wealthy princess Cynisca found herself a participant in the Olympics, thanks to a bit of a loophole. In chariot racing, it was the owner and master of the horses who was considered the official competitor, not the racer (who was usually a slave) or the horses (because they were horses). At the encouragement of her brother, Cynisca entered the tethrippon, a four-horse chariot race, in 396 BCE. She won, then repeated the feat four years later. Although she was not allowed to enter the stadium for the awards ceremony, she did get to place a statue in Zeus's sanctuary, as was the tradition for tethrippon winners at the time. "I declare myself the only woman in all Hellas to have won this crown," reads the inscription she chose.

Cynisca was proud, and rightfully so. She'd found a way to do something no other woman had done before. And even though some suspect her brother only encouraged her to enter in order to make a mockery of the entire process—the point was that wealth, not athletic ability, was the deciding factor in who won chariot races, since more money equaled better horses—Cynisca still pushed the envelope on what a woman could achieve.

She came from Sparta, where things were a little different compared with the rest of Greece. Women in Sparta trained in sports, as long as they were virgins, and even got to compete against one another. Spartan lawgiver Lycurgus was pro strength training for girls, though his logic might not exactly jive with what we think of as feminist today. Philosopher Xenophon said this about his reasoning: "Lycurgus, thinking that the first and foremost function of the freeborn woman was to bear children, ordered that the female should do no less bodybuilding than the male. He thus established contests for the women in footraces and strength, just like those for the men, believing that stronger children come from parents who are both strong."

This was confirmed by biographer Plutarch, who noted that Lycurgus had the girls wrestle, run, and throw the discus and javelin—everything the boys were doing. His goal was to remove softness, daintiness, and effeminacy. In what was considered a risqué practice by most contemporaries, boys and girls exercised together.

This strategy worked. Spartan women were buff, and Plutarch approved of Lycurgus's approach of letting the girls in on the action. "It gave also to womankind a taste of lofty sentiment," he wrote, "for they felt that they, too, had a place in the arena of bravery and ambition."

Brave and ambitious—why shouldn't that be female?

NOT EVERYONE WAS ON BOARD with these ideals. Although Spartan women were well known throughout Greece for their unparalleled beauty (probably an outer reflection of their inner health), Athenian playwright Euripides, for his part, was not a fan:

> No Spartan girl
> could ever live clean even if she wanted.
> They're always out on the street in scanty outfits,
> Making a great display of naked limbs.
> In those they race and wrestle with the boys too—
> Abominable's the word.

For girls to exercise was unclean, but the same criticisms don't seem to have been leveled against boys. In Plato's *Republic*, his teacher, Socrates, said this: "The most ridiculous thing of all will be the sight of women naked in the palaestra, exercising with the men, especially when they are no longer young; they certainly will not be a vision of beauty."

The one-two punch of ageism and sexism is something that would have been nice to leave in ancient times, but how often have you heard a woman's body criticized for not being attractive enough for a swimsuit or whatever "inappropriate" piece of clothing she's chosen to wear, especially once she's left her twenties behind? Plato, to his credit, dismissed the concern, maintaining that men and women should be treated equally. He felt gymnastics, riding, archery, javelin throwing, footraces, and fencing were all appropriate for girls. Eventually, he reasoned, society's biases would disappear. He was right in some ways—there are innumerable women today who are incredible gymnasts, archers, and fencers—but until "You throw like a girl" is a compliment instead of an insult, equal treatment will remain elusive.

While Socrates thought girls exercising alongside boys was ridiculous, he could admit they had athletic skill—to a point. After watching a girl juggle twelve hoops while tumbling, he said her performance helped prove that a woman's nature was not inferior to man's but that women lacked physical strength and judgment. Contradictory much? For a famous thinker, it's maybe not the most airtight argument, but it is a popular one. It's also incredibly frustrating, because even when indisputable skill was displayed right in front of his eyes, he found a way to dismiss it for no evidence-backed reason. The girl's talents challenged a belief he couldn't bear to part with—that males are superior in strength and smarts. Rather than dig a little deeper to try to confront *why* he felt this way and home in on what that feeling was rooted in, Socrates defaulted to the well-worn idea that men are just better, obviously, no explanation necessary.

EVEN IF MOST GREEKS DIDN'T think much of the physical strength of the women in their midst, there was a group of powerful ladies they did find fascinating: the Amazons.

Every Greek hero, from Heracles to Achilles, had to prove himself against these exotic warrior women. Described as equal to men in their fighting abilities, Amazons were said to live in female-only societies, finding men to mate with just once a year, and leaving behind any newborn boys. Rumor had it that they cut off their right breasts in order to shoot an arrow with more precision. They were depicted in Greek art as brave warriors, women to be both feared and respected.

Greek mythology even had an Amazon-like heroine of its own in Atalanta. As a baby, she was abandoned on a mountainside by her father for committing the unforgivable sin of not being born a boy. According to the story, instead of dying, she was nursed to health by a mama bear and later found by a group of hunters. She became quite adept with a bow and a spear and loved to wrestle. When only the fiercest of fighters were recruited for a dangerous expedition to take out the fire-breathing Calydonian Boar, who was wreaking havoc on the community of Calydon, Atalanta was the sole woman invited.

She was doing just fine for herself, but her father insisted she marry—yes, the same loving pops who left her for dead as an infant. She wasn't all that into the idea, so she turned it into a contest. If a man could beat her in a footrace, she'd become his wife. On the plus side, she gave all the contenders a head start. On the minus side, she killed with a spear anyone who failed.

Despite the risk, a whole lot of guys lined up to take their shot, then promptly died. And still, they kept trying. Finally, one was victorious. Hippomenes won out, thanks to a little help from Aphrodite, the goddess of love, who supplied the hopeful suitor with some magic golden apples.

Atalanta was a woman who could give any man a run for his money (or, perhaps more fittingly, a run for his life). Her name comes from the Greek word *atalantos*, which means "equal in weight," presumably a high compliment that she was considered on par with men. As an example, when two centaurs tried to take advantage of her, she killed them. Most stories involving centaurs behaving badly around women ended with a man coming to the rescue, but Atalanta was more than capable of taking care of herself.

While that was impressive, it was also her fatal flaw that she wouldn't accept her prescribed gender role. In the end, it was a man, her misogynistic father, who got to decide if she married. She lost the footrace and the chastity she'd been trying to protect, and once she'd accepted that outcome and was happy with Hippomenes, she and her hubby were turned into lions so that the two could never make love again. (For reasons that aren't completely clear, the Greeks believed lions couldn't mate with one another, only with leopards.) It sends quite the message about the consequences of female independence.

Atalanta was a mythological creation—she was turned into a four-legged animal, after all—and for a long time, scholars have maintained that all Amazons were a figment of imagination in storytelling or perhaps just men mistaken for women. However, there's now evidence that ancient female warriors, aka Amazons, did in fact exist. The Scythians, as they were known to the Greeks, were horse-riding nomads who lived in Eurasia, and both the men and the women were armed and dangerous.

SCYTHIAN REMAINS HAVE BEEN FOUND everywhere from modern-day Bulgaria to Mongolia, buried along with the remnants of weapons such as bows, arrows, daggers, spears, and sling stones. Their bones are marred by the signs of repeated breakings and healings, arrowheads still embedded in some. Until recently, archaeologists assumed the skeletons surrounded by all these sharp accoutrements belonged to men. But advances in science and DNA testing have revealed that not all of those skeletons are men; in some archaeological digs, more than a quarter of the unearthed Scythians are women buried with the implements of a fighter. Adrienne Mayor, author of *The Amazons,* told *National Geographic,* "If you think about it, a woman on a horse with a bow, trained since childhood, can be just as fast and as deadly as a boy or man."

For a bit of Amazon myth busting, there's no evidence that there were entire societies of women warriors who shunned men. They did not maim young boys, and it's not likely that they were cutting off their right breasts in order to shoot an arrow better. The way they held their bows wasn't all that close to their chests, and common sense tells us that archery wouldn't be easier with a missing boob. (The mistaken notion of self-mutilation that's been perpetuated in pop culture probably originated from an erroneous etymological interpretation of *Amazon*, as the *a-* prefix means "without" in Greek, and *mazos* kinda sorta sounds like *mastos*, which means "breast.")

However, they just might have sent their boys off to other tribes, not to get rid of them so they could keep the sisterhood strong but because sending children to be raised by other tribes was a common practice in antiquity that fostered good relations and helped keep incest at bay. In most Greek households, girls were considered a burden, less valuable than boys, but among the Scythians, there was equality—all children learned to ride a horse, shoot an arrow, and find sustenance.

The women traveled by horseback, hunted for food, fought for glory, chose their partners, and exercised autonomy. And they did this all while wearing pants, considered barbaric by the tunic-sporting Greeks. This gave them the freedom to move comfortably, no small luxury. "The Greeks were both fascinated and appalled by such independent women," Mayor said. "They were so different from their wives and daughters. Yet there was a fascination. They were captivated by them. Pictures of Amazons on vase paintings always show them as beautiful, active, spirited, courageous, and brave." Through these depictions, Mayor believes, there's a clear "yearning and desire for some kind of resolution to the tension between 'Yes, we want them as our companions,' and 'We couldn't possibly, because we have to control our own women.' " That confusing push and pull, from admiration to derision, continued many years after the final Scythians rode off into the sunset.

• • •

OVER IN ANCIENT ROME, JUST across the Mediterranean Sea, there's evidence that athletics were an option for at least some of the girls. In the twelfth century CE, a mudslide covered Sicily's Villa Romana del Casale, likely the residence of a Roman senatorial aristocrat from the fourth century, and the dirt kept what lay beneath remarkably well preserved.

When archaeologists unearthed one room in the 1950s, they called the mosaic inside "The Bikini Girls," for the images of ladies in small tops and bottoms appeared to them like some type of bikini-clad beauty pageant. A modern lens tells a different story: these are sports bras and booty shorts perfect for working out; the laurel crowns they receive are prizes for winning athletic competitions,

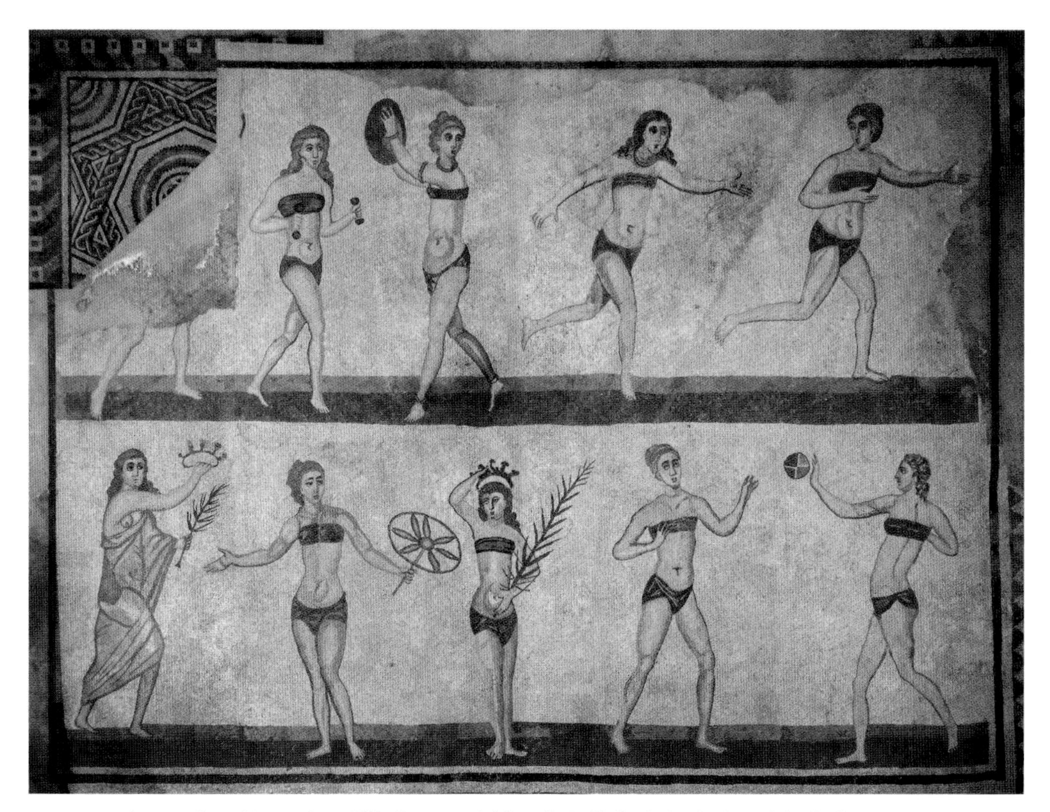

A centuries-old mosaic at Villa Romana del Casale in Sicily, Italy, depicts girls playing sports.

not for smiling prettily. The ten young women are depicted performing activities such as jumping with weights in their hands, throwing a discus, tossing a ball, and running.

Historians believe that by the time the mosaic was created, some women had been playing sports in ancient Rome for hundreds of years. In addition to the running, throwing, and ball games depicted in the mosaic, these women practiced gladiatorial combat, acrobatics, and swimming.

IF THIS SOUNDS AS IF women had plenty of opportunities for sport in ancient times, that might be because I've zoomed way in, combing through history for any and every mention of girls developing guns. Hundreds of men make up the victory lists that have survived, while only a handful of women appear. "For each vase depicting women in sport-like activities, there are many, many more showing men in athletic activities or in palaestra scenes," writes Betty Spears, a former professor of sport studies. "The history of women's sport is based on a very few facts and the history of men's sport on abundant data. . . . Generally, women's sport was perceived as insignificant except for a few highly skilled women."

Basically, our ancient female counterparts' role in the realm of athletics was a blip on the radar. And while we don't have all the artifacts from ancient times to know everything that went on, what does survive shows that women's efforts to pursue strength—and society's attempt to prevent such efforts—go way back to the dawn of Western civilization. Considerable attention was paid to keeping women stuck indoors, and when they were allowed to participate in athletics, it was not often at a high level. Many girls who wanted to engage in sports were in a no-win situation—criticized when they were like the boys and playing the same games yet also criticized for not being as good at said games. Remember, as Euripides said of these girls, "abominable's the word." The boys were always the measuring stick, the girls never quite there. Their role was in the home, not in the arena of bravery and ambition. Everything the Greeks believed about being of sound mind and body extended to only half the population.

Perhaps it sounds a little familiar? The physical rights of women still don't equal those of men, and in some ways and places, they're regressing. Male lawmakers make decisions on behalf of women, as Atalanta's father did, under the guise that they know best. How many impossibly destructive boars does a woman have to take down to prove that she's fit to make choices for herself?

Lycurgus was on to something when he said that strong fathers *and* mothers lead to a stronger society. But there's more to it than just passing on genes to the next generation.

A strong woman might compete in a sprint, train a champion boxer, win a horse race, be equally happy married or single, or know how to fend for herself—and who wouldn't want a society stacked with capable, inspirational people like that?

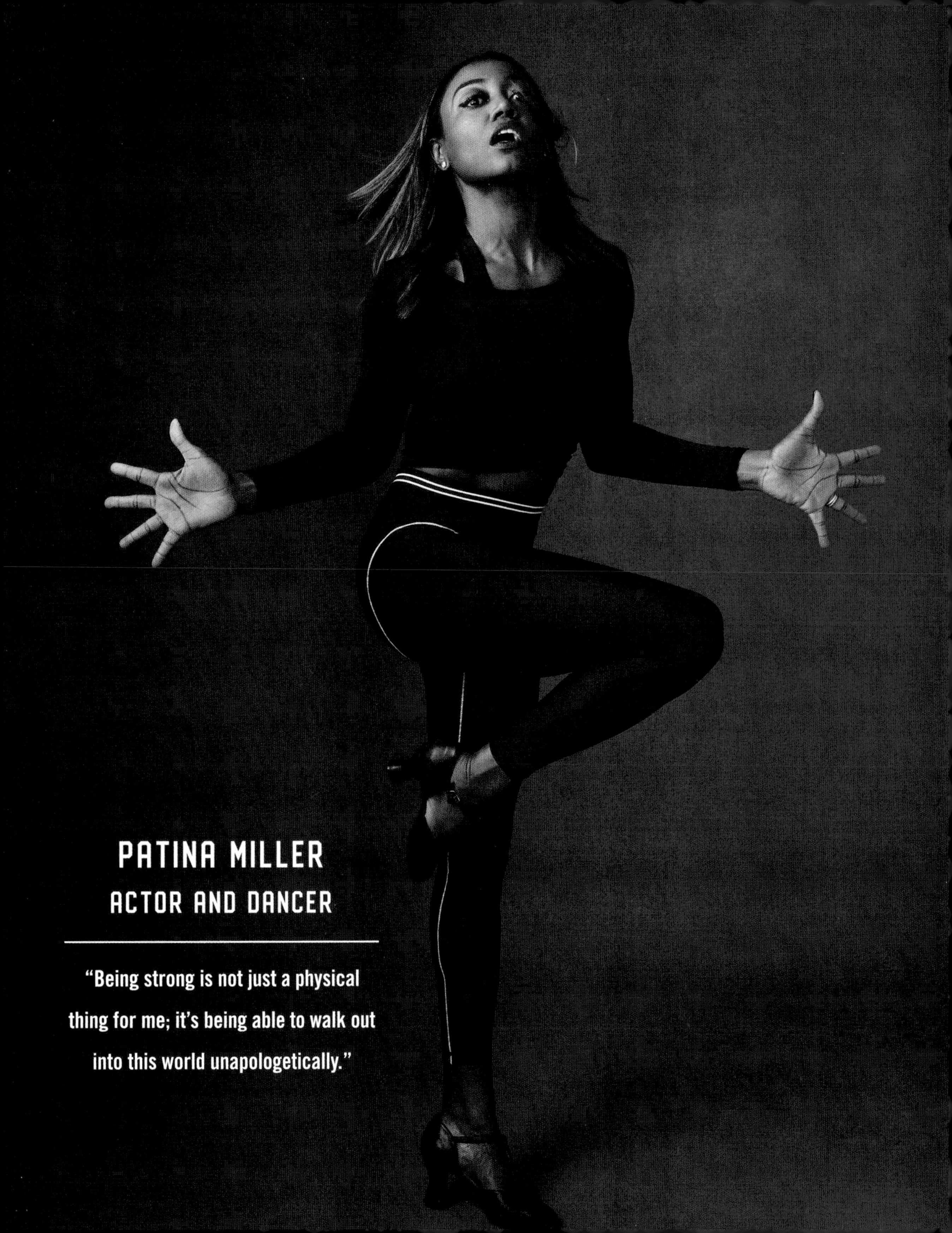

PATINA MILLER
ACTOR AND DANCER

"Being strong is not just a physical thing for me; it's being able to walk out into this world unapologetically."

CHAPTER 2

THE OUTLIERS:

VICTORIAN-ERA WOMEN WHO WALKED ON THE WILD SIDE

When Queen Victoria ascended to the British throne in 1837 at the tender age of eighteen, most people expected her to be a weak, ineffectual ruler. She was young, shy, small in stature, and plain-looking. Even her name was ridiculous, not regal like Anne or Mary. Some thought it might be the end of the monarchy. When the archbishop of Canterbury and the lord chamberlain arrived early in the morning upon the passing of her uncle to inform the princess of her new role, her governess prepared smelling salts to revive her, in the likely case that she would faint. She didn't need them.

Spanning sixty-three years, the Victorian era (named for that very queen) became known as one of the most iconic periods of history, boasting a list of world-altering developments: the first telegraph, the Industrial Revolution, and the rise of the middle class, to name just a few.

Until she became queen, Victoria had to share a room with her domineering mother, and she wasn't even allowed to walk down a set of stairs alone. But Victoria was strong and stubborn, showing she wasn't the delicate flower she had been raised to be. After getting the news that she had inherited the throne, she had the opportunity to assert herself for the very first time—which she used to request one hour to herself, a luxury she'd never before had. She then jumped into her reign ready to lead. Queen Victoria was apprehensive about marriage yet ended up proposing to her cousin Albert. She let him know in no uncertain terms that he was not to "boss her about" and that she did not want to have many children, and yet she did acquiesce to quite a bit of bossing and ended up giving birth to five girls and four boys.

The queen was a study in contrasts, much like her eponymous era itself. This was a time when modesty, manners, family life, and sexual propriety mattered very much, but it was also a time when children were put to work in factories doing dangerous jobs and when prostitution was rampant.

A woman's relationship to strength was just as conflicted. Like their ancient female counterparts, Victorian women were mostly relegated to matters of hearth and home. They were expected to lace up their waists in tight corsets, to be prim and proper, to sip tea and fall victim to fainting spells because of their delicate constitution. These expectations could go a long way in fashioning women's behavior. On the other hand, in a period of rapid change, women were pushing the boundaries of their preconceived abilities the world over. Across the ocean in the United States, schools were increasingly adding physical education programs for girls, more than a quarter of all new bicycles in 1896 went to women, and when people showed up in droves to watch the country's first spectator sport, ladies had a chance to play the starring role.

THE SPORT WAS CALLED PEDESTRIANISM, and it was quite the craze in the United States in the 1870s and '80s, after starting in England and Scotland. While most participants were men, a fair number of women's contests were held, too. In the U.K., the sport had been practiced by girls and women since at least the 1820s, if not earlier. It was an opportunity to earn money, fame, and ink in sporting newspapers, another rare chance for a woman.

Pedestrian events took place both indoors and outdoors to see just how far athletes could walk. They might journey from point A to point B—say, Portland, Maine, to Chicago, Illinois—or, more likely, walk around a track in an arena, racking up a certain amount of mileage within a certain time constraint. Six-day extravaganzas, from Monday morning to Saturday night, became standard, given that public entertainment on Sundays was frowned upon or even outright banned.

The best walkers vaulted into the celebrity stratosphere, their images splashed on cigarette trading cards, their pursuits sponsored by corporations, their gaits and strategies analyzed and dissected the way we discuss a quarterback's stats today. Even President Chester A. Arthur was a fan.

Of the women, the U.K.'s Ada Anderson was particularly good. She trained as any serious athlete would, first by seeking out a mentor, champion racewalker William Gale, who taught her how to walk really far on very little sleep. The sleep part was key—while endurance was crucial, of course, it was nearly impossible to succeed unless one was a polyphasic sleeper, someone who could sleep in short blocks as opposed to all at once. ("Short blocks" in this case means just a handful of minutes at a time, a few zzz's short of the eight consecutive hours most of us like to get.)

In her debut event, Anderson walked 1,000 half miles in 1,000 half hours (500 miles in a three-week period), resting no longer than twenty minutes at a time. After trying singing, acting, performing as a circus clown, and running concert halls—all pursuits in which she failed to excel—she had finally found her thing. Once she became a dominant force in England and Wales, she set her sights on the U.S. pedestrianism market.

Her manager tried to set up an attempt of 2,700 quarter miles in 2,700 quarter hours (675 miles in about twenty-eight days) in New York, but the request was denied. "The woman can never accomplish the feat, nor can any other woman;

it is simply an impossibility," said William Kissam Vanderbilt, who owned the arena then called Gilmore's Garden, which would become Madison Square Garden.

Anderson went to the newly constructed Mozart Garden instead, a small venue in Brooklyn where the track was so short that she had to walk it seven times just to get to a quarter mile. Vanderbilt was not wrong in thinking it was a difficult task, but underestimating Anderson was a miscalculation. As many as four thousand people a *day* came to watch her walk the track in her quest to circle it 18,900 times, and the event proved so popular that by the final day, people were paying two dollars for reserved seating (up from twenty-five cents). Police began forbidding the sale of any additional tickets, since Mozart Garden had reached capacity. "The little hall is calculated to hold about 1,000 persons comfortably," the *New York Times* reported, "but double that number and perhaps more were packed into it like sardines last night, and wedged so closely together that any movement save of the head and arms was impossible."

Of the huge numbers of people streaming through the doors to see her walk, the *Times* reported, "These crowds are largely composed of women, and of these no small portion are ladies." Ladies were described in the *Brooklyn Eagle* as those who wore sealskin dresses and hats overflowing with feathers, always accompanied by a charming escort. Women were, apparently, a different, non-sealskin-wearing sort.

With the squished, enthusiastic crowd behind her—men, women, children, *and* ladies—Anderson accomplished her goal and did it in style, singing to the audience and completing the final quarter mile in just 2:37.75, the fastest of all the seven-lap stretches. For her efforts, she earned a cool $8,000, which would be more than $200,000 in today's dollars. Afterward, she sipped port wine while being lauded for showing the women of Brooklyn just what they could achieve.

It was difficult, though, for the average woman to imagine herself exerting as much energy as Anderson did. That's partly because walking for weeks on end with no real sleep is kind of nuts in any era for any person, but that aside, women of this time were viewed as the morally superior but physically inferior sex. Bed rest was the prescription of the day for any "nervous illness" a woman might have, which kept her weak and isolated from family and friends for weeks at a time. As basic physics teaches us, an object at rest stays at rest. Spend all your time resting, and it's pretty hard to get moving. At the time, walking two blocks was considered plenty of exercise for an American woman.

But Madame Anderson, as she called herself, proved that womanhood and weakness were not inextricably linked. "The idea, as general as it is venerable, that a woman cannot, by reason of her sex, endure as much as a man, is exploded, and to Madame Anderson is due the overthrow of the mistaken notion," the *Brooklyn Daily Eagle* wrote.

She went on to achieve more in the sport, including 351 miles in six days and 804 miles in 500 hours. Her accomplishments opened women's eyes. Instead of assuming their bodies were always on the verge of falling apart, as they'd been told by the male medical establishment, perhaps they could use activity as a way to better health. Maybe, just maybe, they weren't as frail as they'd been led to believe.

Anderson wasn't just different from the average Victorian woman; she even set herself apart from other "pedestriennes." While many walked in long petticoats and were more overtly ladylike, Anderson dared to bare her knees. When she addressed a crowd, her speeches were straightforward and confident, not laced with humility. She'd been married twice but spent much of her life single, and she had no children. Her build was muscular, and her face was described in papers as "slightly masculine." Despite coming across as unconventional, Anderson won people over with her expressive eyes, robust health, and charismatic

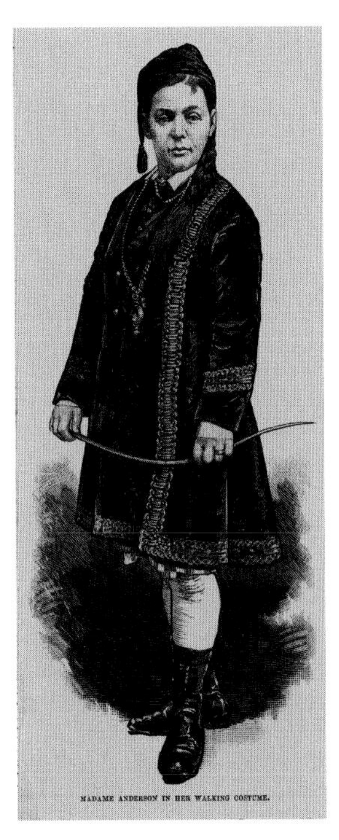

Ada Anderson strikes a regal pose before her historic walk in Brooklyn's Mozart Garden.

presence (she was quite a prankster, using a burnt cork to mark the faces of crowd members who fell asleep at her contests). Her stride was described as graceful, swaying, "poetry of motion."

Still, as impressive as Anderson's athleticism was, and as much as she may have challenged the notion of women as fragile, her accomplishments were in no way universally revered. People even found moral grounds on which to object to the sport—she and many other pedestrians walked on Sundays, gambling was involved, and they seemed to be putting their health at risk by going to such extremes. Anderson tried to mitigate these effects by extolling the virtues of exercise and offering a special entrance for families at her walks, so they could avoid seeing any unsavory displays such as gambling. She was also sure to thank God for her abilities, a good step toward heading off arguments of immorality.

Yet even as women proved that their walking bouts were just as entertaining as men's and that they could go the distance, there were still powerful forces at work to maintain the status quo. Health activist Dr. John Harvey Kellogg, of cereal fame, was an outspoken critic of women testing themselves this way. A woman was "generally less graceful and naturally less skillful in the use of the extremities than [a] man, and hence less fitted for athletic sports and feats requiring great dexterity," he wrote, adding that "nothing could be much more inhuman" than a pedestrian contest with women. Another doctor posited that the pelvis shape changed during puberty, making the knees closer together, and that was what led to the "awkward" running gait that only women possessed. This bodily analysis emphasizing a woman's natural lack of physical prowess came from doctors, in a profession that was highly respected, so these claims were put forth with more than a little authority.

"Peculiar" hips and limbs aside, pedestrianism wasn't the only women's sport with mixed feelings attached to it in the second half of the nineteenth century. While this style of marathon walking has fallen by the wayside, another sport emerged soon after that's probably a bit more familiar: basketball. Just a handful of years after James Naismith invented it, women were ready to officially take their shot.

ON THE DAY THAT STANFORD UNIVERSITY was set to play the University of California, Berkeley, the Armory in San Francisco was packed with more than seven hundred female fans. Men were not allowed—the Berkeley team didn't think it was proper for gentlemen to see them in bloomers, sweating—but that only stoked male curiosity. They climbed the venue's roof and peered through the windows while women inside batted them away with sticks.

It was April 1896, and this was the first time two women's college teams would officially go head-to-head in the emerging sport. While basketball had been developed for men, it was quickly adapted for women—in fact, Naismith himself thought it was an ideal sport for the fairer sex. To make it more female-friendly, a physical education instructor at Smith College named Senda Berenson changed up the rules, dividing the court into thirds and requiring the players to remain within their assigned sections. This prevented excessive running and kept the focus on cooperation. You could dribble the ball a maximum of three times, could hold it for no more than five seconds, and were prohibited from snatching it from anyone's hands.

The rules, however, didn't stop the players from being scrappy. Wearing bloomers, long-sleeved sweaters, and black stockings, they weren't afraid to hustle. "The fighting was hard and the playing good," the *San Francisco Examiner* reported. "The girls jumped, scrambled and fell over one another on the floor. But they didn't mind it. They were up as quick as a flash, chasing after the ball again."

Coming in, the Berkeley women looked as if they might be the team to beat. They were taller and stronger and, according to a reporter, had more-gorgeous hair. (Stanford's was "curly for the most part and disordered about the ears.")

This might not be the hard-hitting coverage we'd expect today, but it was incredibly detailed. The newspapers took this game seriously, a sign that they believed female athletes were worth the column inches.

Unfortunately for Berkeley, impressive tresses do not automatically make for good hook shots. "The two girls they had depended on to score for them missed the basket repeatedly, to their own confusion and the undoing of the team," the *San Francisco Chronicle* reported.

Stanford missed plenty, too, but managed to put up the first point (each basket counted for one point back then) before knocking their hoop off-kilter. A janitor and his assistant came to fix it, conspicuously becoming the only men in the room. Some of the Berkeley athletes let out muffled screams and ran to a corner to hide.

After the diversion, Berkeley answered with a point of its own, tying it up, and it remained a tightly contested matchup from there on out.

Ultimately, Stanford prevailed. Final score: 2-1.

This was just one example among the collegiate crowd of a new idea that was taking hold: women playing sports not just for health or recreational reasons but for performance and competition. In 1898, Abbie Carter Goodloe wrote in *Scribner's* magazine of college rowers: "In their dark blouses and bloomers, the muscular young rowers of today present a very different appearance from those of other years, when the formation of a crew was almost a social affair, and those who composed it were elevated chiefly for their good looks." (Prior to this, female rowers were judged based not on whose boat was fastest but on their form and grace.) And at women-only Wellesley College, a writer in the yearbook gushed about the basketball team: "The grimy and generally disheveled appearance of the players, as they emerge from the fray, fills our athletic souls with pride."

After the Stanford women were victorious, the team returned to Palo Alto to much fanfare, complete with cheering students and a marching band. You would think this was a victory for women's sports as well, but once again, the pendulum swung the other way, powered by public opinion. By the end of 1899, Stanford had discontinued women's intercollegiate team sports, citing health concerns and unpleasant publicity as reasons. Competitive sports, administrators said, were too dangerous, with too high a risk of corrupting the souls of young women. Men's sports continued.

In actuality, the souls of the first basketball players didn't seem to be harmed in any way. These women went on to be quite successful—they became doctors, teachers, a nurse, and a college professor, to name a few. But no matter how many times women proved themselves, it often wasn't enough. The basketball team was, by all accounts, hardworking, popular, and deserving of the opportunity to play, an opportunity they wouldn't get again at Stanford and many other colleges for more than six decades.

THIS SEESAW OF EXPERT AND public opinion was nothing new. There were advocates for women like the influential educator Catharine Beecher, sister of famous abolitionist Harriet Beecher Stowe, who believed girls should be taught a robust range of academic subjects, as boys were, from Latin and history to algebra and logic. Beecher championed physical education, too, introducing calisthenics in her classrooms at the Hartford Female Seminary in 1824. "Confinement to one position, for a great length of time, tends to weaken the muscles thus strained," she wrote. "This shows the evil of confining young children to their seats, in the schoolroom, so much and so long as is often done."

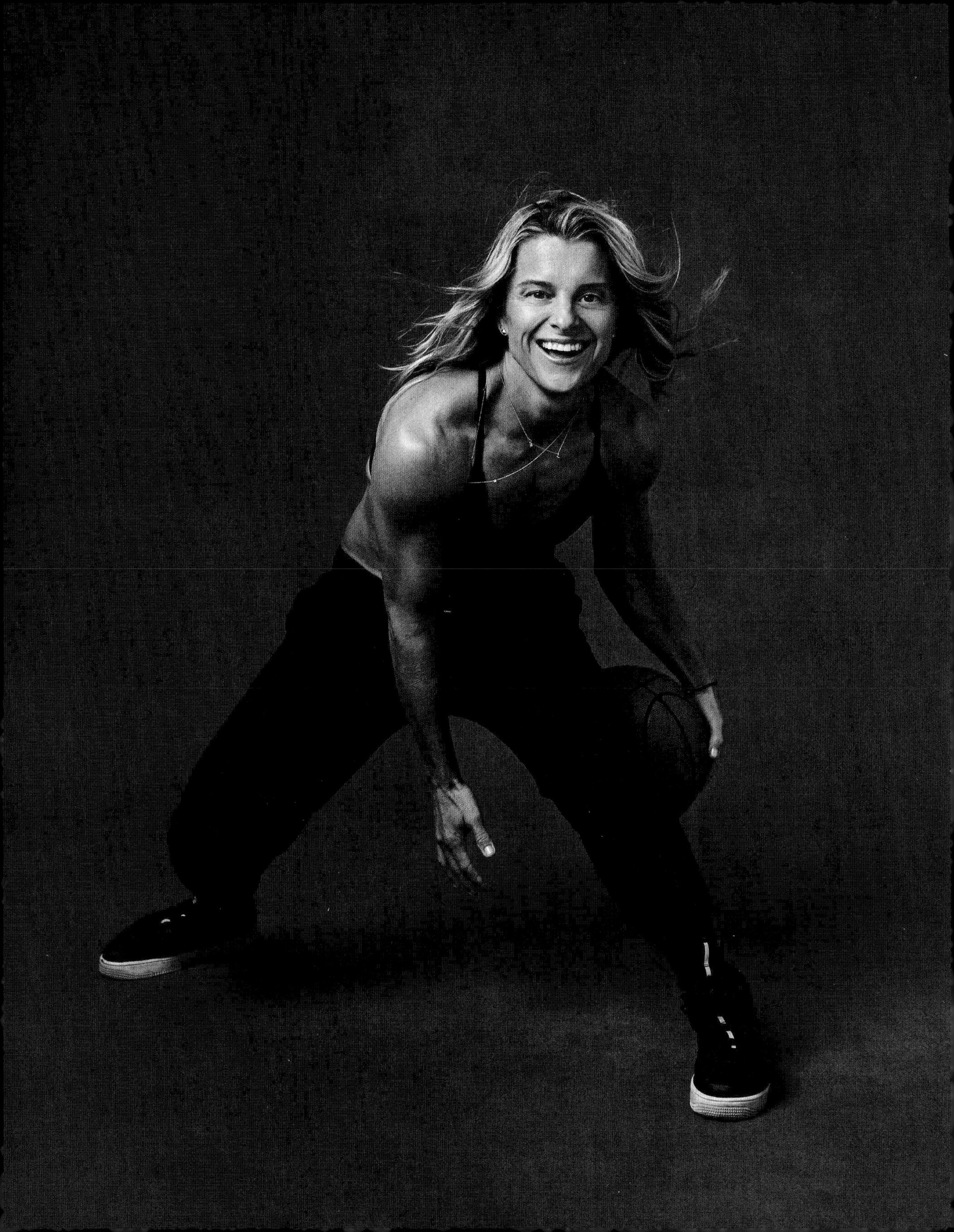

"COURAGE DOESN'T ALWAYS ROAR. SOMETIMES IT'S A QUIET VOICE AT THE END OF THE DAY SAYING, 'YOU CAN TRY AGAIN TOMORROW.' "

HOLLY RILINGER

BASKETBALL PLAYER AND TRAINER

Her grandniece, prominent writer Charlotte Perkins Gilman, was deeply influenced by these teachings, and she delighted in her own physical abilities. "I could vault and jump, go up a knotted rope, walk on my hands under a ladder, kick as high as my head, and revel in the flying rings," she wrote. As she strengthened her body, she felt she was strengthening her character. She called the 1879 muscle-building manual *How to Get Strong and How to Stay So* by William Blaikie her "Atalanta guidebook."

The book's author, Blaikie, believed women who were fit could "spend life with an appreciation and zest too often unknown by the weak woman" and urged them not to be afraid of the shape muscles bring. In an 1899 update to his hit book, Blaikie quoted a doctor from Ohio as saying: "Any muscle, well developed, is beautiful; muscular lines are lines of beauty everywhere. I have yet to hear admiration of a lady's arm that has not good biceps and triceps under its coating of feminine adipose; and as to the forearm, the most beautiful specimens in flesh and blood that I know of are the forearms of pianistes, who have muscles of steel from wrist to elbow."

Marriage, pregnancy, and postpartum depression kept Gilman away from the gym for a long while. When she finally returned, she wrote in her diary, "Happy to the verge of idiocy." Gilman loved feeling like an athlete, and her husband admired that quality in her, too—until she wanted to divorce him. Then he complained to newspapers that she'd taken fitness too far. "She became very muscular!" he lamented.

IN CONTRAST TO THE PROGRESSIVE ideas proposed by Beecher and Blaikie, there were other theories we can look back on now with amusement, but in truth, they demonstrate the use of disinformation to keep women in their place. For example, *American Farmer* magazine warned women in 1827 that if they exercised, they were quite likely to grow small tumors on their ankle joints, much like young horses that were worked too hard did, and *Harper's Weekly* in 1860 shared the harrowing tale of a "lady-skater" who tied her laces too tight and needed to have her foot amputated. Fear has always been a handy tool to keep someone in her place.

Many girls longed to do more, to lace up their skates just tight enough to glide with abandon. German Hedwig Dohm, who was known as one of the first feminist thinkers to propose that gender roles were a result of socialization, not biology, wrote in a semiautobiographical novel: "The boys were lucky. They did gymnastics. They exercised. They were allowed to romp around freely in the streets and squares. Snow and ice was theirs in the winter, the lake in the summer. We girls didn't do gymnastics, we didn't swim, we didn't row. We weren't allowed to have snowball fights, not even to skate."

And so they busied themselves with needlework and other similar activities, and "grace" was considered a legitimate health goal. They were often warned not to exert themselves too much. "Fresh air is absolutely essential to keep one in health, but most women get sufficient exercise in moving about their households, and a long walk does not bring sufficient compensation for the fatigue it causes," wrote Elisabeth Robinson Scovil in 1896's *Preparation for Motherhood*, adding that lying in a hammock during the summer was more beneficial than being on one's feet.

The Victorians urged against physical activity in particular during one's period, and the young women at Vassar College were not supposed to go up or down stairs during the first two days of their menstrual cycles. In the Victorian mind, energy was a finite resource, and once it was gone, there was no replenishing it, so rest was needed to get through womanly tasks such as menstruating, giving birth, and breastfeeding. If you didn't rest, you were risking the health of future generations, a selfish choice indeed. (Menstruation and its relation to fitness has remained full of mystery since then—and a method of keeping women out of sports. In the late 1990s, the British Boxing Board of Control said that PMS made women too "unstable" to box, and in 2016, after Chinese swimmer Fu Yuanhui made headlines at the Olympics for explaining that she appeared to be in pain because she had gotten her period the night before, many expressed disbelief through social media that a woman could even swim during her period, genuinely wondering how the pool didn't turn red.)

Energy as a finite resource also applied to intellectual capabilities. If you exerted yourself too much while riding a horse or playing a game of tennis, you were limiting your academic potential in a way that you might not be able to recover from. Did you want A's on your tests or a proficient backhand?

Despite these discouraging messages, as the 1800s went on, more and more schools offered some kind of physical education for girls. Indian clubs, which resemble an elongated bowling pin, were among the common implements for working out. A combination of Indian clubs, light dumbbells, and weighted wands formed the basis of a gymnastics program created in the 1860s by Dr. Dio Lewis that was popular in Northeastern schools for women. Lewis, who believed that America's future pivoted on the "great woman revolution," was against corsets and believed boys and girls should exercise together, preferably with a little music playing so that it would be fun. In his 1871 etiquette book, *Our Girls*, he threw serious shade at shoemakers for their strange insistence on making footwear for girls that ran too narrow, with soles too flimsy to last outdoors. He wrote, "Some people seem, somehow, to suppose that girls do not really step on the ground, but that, in some sort of spiritual way, they pass along just above the damp, unclean earth. But, as a matter of fact, girls do step on the ground just like boys. I have frequently walked behind them to test this point, and have noticed that when the ground is soft, they make tracks, and thus demonstrate the existence of an actual, material body."

Women were often criticized for not walking as elegantly as men, but it's kind of hard to be a paragon of efficient movement with your foot squished into a shoe half the width it should be, a common problem at the time. In the absence of constrictive clothing, who knew what one could achieve?

IN THE GILDED AGE—FROM THE late 1860s through the mid-1890s, when the unprecedented growth of big business led to American "royalty" (that is, absurdly rich families who put their wealth on display)—some sports fared better than others in terms of public acceptance for women. High-class sports such as tennis, croquet, and archery were all respected, for one simple reason: the dress code. These sports' cumbersome and elaborate costumes, which branded competitors as feminine, allowed them to enter the mainstream. It could be a stealthy method of packaging progress and simultaneously a real hindrance to the actual execution of one's sport.

The question of just what women should wear while exercising—and while doing anything, really—was always a hot topic. Lewis advocated loose pants and a jacket, a fairly radical suggestion. The Stanford and Berkeley basketball players of 1896 had their uniforms described by the press in painstaking detail, down to how they were wearing their hair and the ribbons on their sweaters. Madame Anderson, who walked away with people's hearts, also had her outfits dissected in detail—something reporters didn't focus on quite so much with male pedestrians. The initial uniform during her historic feat in Brooklyn, for example, consisted of "black velvet knee breeches, and a loose flowing robe of blue and scarlet cloth, embroidered with white, descending just far enough to allow the free exercise of the body. On her feet were stout, loose leather shoes, topped by stockings of flaming scarlet. Her rounded limbs were inclosed in silver tights."

At the 1900 Paris Olympics, women were allowed to participate for the first time, with options of golf, tennis, sailing, croquet, and equestrian events. They wore ankle-length dresses with long sleeves and high necks, accessorized with heeled shoes. To say their performance was hindered compared with the men—in shorts and cotton T-shirts—is an understatement.

When women performing in a gymnastics exhibition at the 1912 Stockholm Olympics dared to wear knee-length skirts, they were chastised for being unladylike. U.S. female swimmers weren't allowed to take part in these Games over concerns that the thigh-length wool swimsuits weren't nearly modest enough. Despite sports slowly gaining acceptance for women, participation was often dependent on whether their outfits conformed to the standards of what women should wear—standards largely created so that they wouldn't incite lust from the men around them—performance be damned.

Decades later, clothing remained of utmost importance for the female athlete. It played a central role in the popularity of the All-American Girls Professional Baseball League when it debuted in the 1940s. The subject of the popular 1992 movie *A League of Their Own*, the league mandated that players wear a feminine, short-skirted, flared tunic in pastel shades with satin shorts underneath.

The league's handbook contained good information about living a healthy, balanced lifestyle, but it also required players to adhere strictly to a "femininity principle." That meant wearing skirts and makeup, keeping their hair long, and attending evening charm school. They were given beauty kits to help keep their appearance as pleasing as possible and were required to apply lipstick—"with moderate taste"—at all times. Bob haircuts were grounds for dismissal, as one player found out the hard way.

This marketing strategy seemed to work. The league drew more than 900,000 fans at its peak in 1948. Would it have become as popular if the players hadn't presented this gender-conforming image? Perhaps not.

The baseball league's uniforms were far from the last to emphasize a certain feminine standard. Female figure skaters were required by the International Skating Union to wear skirts until 2004, and sporting bikini bottoms no wider than six centimeters on the sides was an International Volleyball Federation rule in beach volleyball until 2012. That same year, women's boxing debuted at the Olympics, and the International Boxing Association mandated that all competitors wear skirts in the ring, before backing down in the face of enormous backlash and adding shorts as an option.

Certain sports were able to make strides behind a curtain of femininity, but putting the focus on things like lipstick shades and the size of bikini bottoms minimized the fact that these women were real athletes. Even today, instead of being able to wear what's best for a particular sport, they may be asked to wear what's best for the viewer. While micromanaging uniforms can be a means to an end for attracting attention, as it was in the All-American Girls Professional Baseball League, it is always a way to highlight (or even exploit) female athletes for their sex and not their skill.

CLOTHES WERE JUST ONE WAY the women of the 1800s were inhibited from earning respect and reaching their full physical potential. Outfitting them in restrictive corsets and too-small shoes only served to reinforce the idea that their movements didn't match those of men.

It's true that they probably didn't walk with the same gait or toss a basketball with the same arc—this much is clear—but what wasn't being questioned was why men's movements were considered the standard. Wide hips are different from narrow hips, but they're neither inferior nor superior. Those kinds of physiological differences—sometimes magnified by the clothing worn—were used as ammunition to make women's physical abilities feel lesser or even nonexistent. "The woman's desire to be on a level of competition with man and to assume his duties is, I am sure, making mischief," wrote Charlotte Perkins Gilman's doctor, who prescribed her the rest cure and told her to live as domestic a life as possible. "She is physiologically other than the man."

Even a woman as powerful as Queen Victoria was worn down by the constraints of her role as a woman. Throughout her nine pregnancies, she became more and more dependent on her husband, Prince Albert. At first, she resented losing some of her power to him, but eventually, she concluded that "we women are not *made* for governing." The low expectations of women likely led to underachieving and a fair amount of opportunities not taken. When they were able to exceed what was thought possible, as the Stanford and Berkeley basketball players did, their opportunities might vanish. It didn't help how mixed the messages were; should one believe the books that advocated active hobbies or the ones that said lounging in a hammock was exercise aplenty?

And yet in the face of all this, women were starting to get a taste of how strength felt—and they liked it. Trailblazers such as Ada Anderson set out to prove that you could carve your own path, one that involved extraordinary achievement physically, mentally, and even economically.

"Her physical powers are the admiration of physicians, and her muscular strength is something to rejoice over," one reporter said of Anderson. "Women are so universally delicate and hyper-nervous that the spectacle of a woman of grand physique is an inspiring one, particularly when with it is associated an intelligent and cultivated mind."

In Anderson's time, there was a gulf between what women were *told* they could do, what they *actually* could do, and what they *believed* they could do. Through Anderson's articulate speeches, clever personality, and unmatched endurance, she proved that women could set big physical goals and achieve them—and they didn't have to worry that all their energy was permanently draining away, robbing them of intellectual capacity as they pursued a stronger body.

"When I first began my walk I asked the ladies for their presence," Anderson said at Mozart Garden. "I think from the number of ladies who have come that they are satisfied. It is good for women to see how much a woman can endure."

But it wasn't just about enduring. As Anderson briskly demonstrated, pushing physical limits wasn't only about gritting through a tough task but about finding enjoyment, self-confidence, and pride in one's ability to do so. Walking in a circle may have appeared futile to some (and, oh, the blisters), but instead of going nowhere fast, Anderson was really marching toward progress.

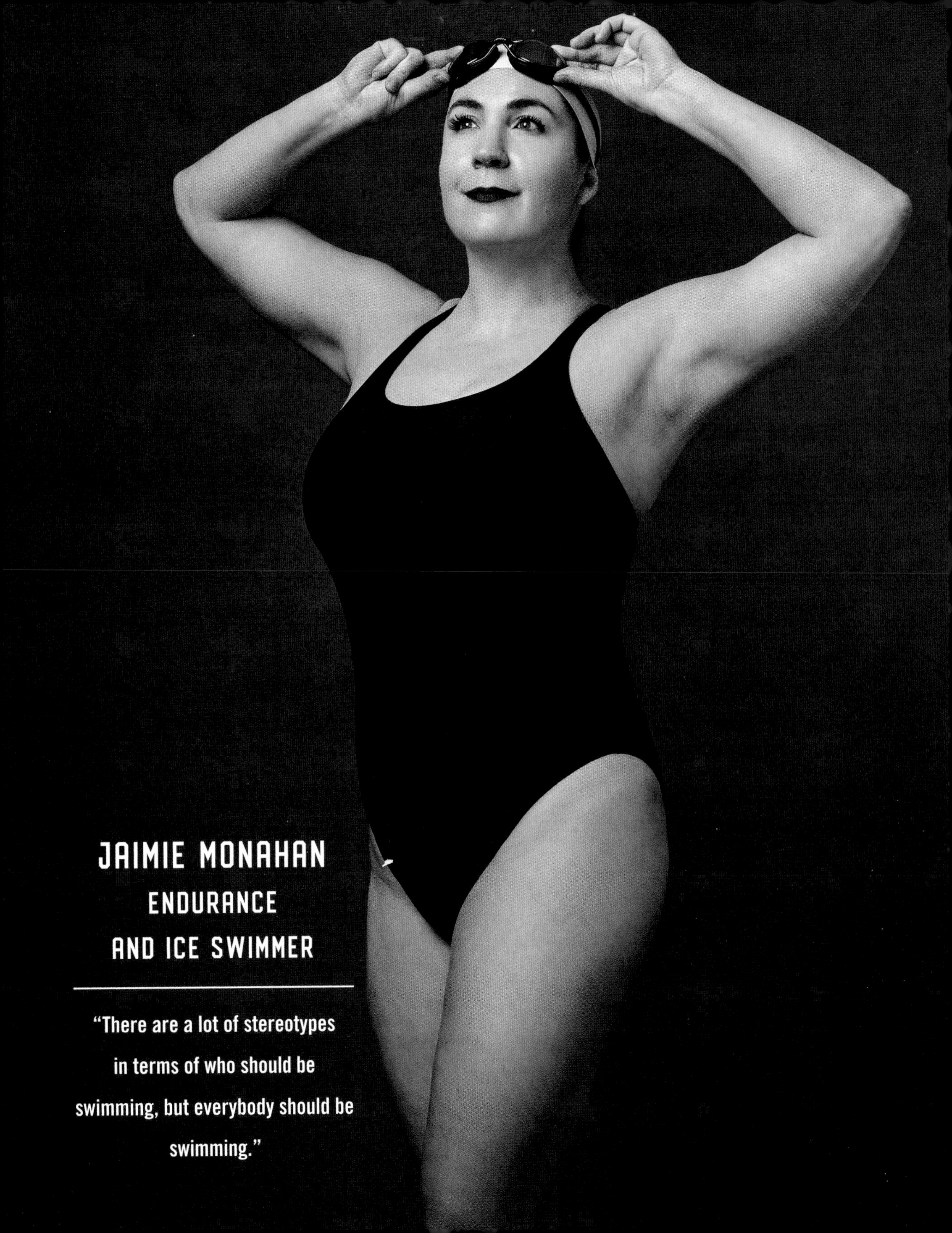

JAIMIE MONAHAN
ENDURANCE AND ICE SWIMMER

"There are a lot of stereotypes in terms of who should be swimming, but everybody should be swimming."

CHAPTER 3

SINK OR SWIM:
STRENGTH AS A MEANS OF SURVIVAL

Sometimes when we think of strength, we focus on the surface results, such as winning a game, as the Stanford basketball players did, or making a lot of money, as Ada Anderson accomplished with her long-distance walking. There's deeper meaning, of course, to the communication skills and improved self-esteem that result from being part of a team or the autonomy that comes from making one's own money. Those types of benefits contribute to living a good life, but sometimes strength is vital to living any life at all.

One of the deadliest events in New York City (second only to September 11, 2001) happened in large part because girls were rarely taught to swim in the early 1900s.

At the time, swimming struck many as masculine, since water sports in general were considered a male domain. There was also that pesky problem surrounding what to wear rearing its head again. The modesty of the times meant swimsuits were made of seven to ten yards of fabric: wool tights, knee-length bloomers, a sailor-style blouse with balloon sleeves, a belt, a full skirt, and swimming shoes or boots. Wool and flannel were the recommended fabrics for swimwear, thanks to their ability to insulate from the cold but not so much their buoyancy when wet. It doesn't take much imagination to realize how heavy that would all be when soaked through.

Would-be swimmers were quite literally constrained by the clothes they wore. The suits worked fine for frolicking along the beach, maybe dipping a toe in the water, but they certainly weren't ideal for any kind of actual horizontal-in-the-water swimming. Many women were afraid their long skirts would tangle around their legs and drown them—not irrational in the least—consequently, they avoided the problem by never learning to swim in the first place.

All of that set the stage for June 15, 1904. The *General Slocum,* a sidewheel passenger steamboat, was chartered by St. Mark's Evangelical Lutheran Church for an annual end-of-school trip from the East Village to Long Island, where a picnic awaited. It was a Wednesday morning, and the majority of the passengers were German-American women and children—kids went for free, so it made sense for moms to bring the entire family. Shortly after leaving the dock, a fire broke out in the forward section of the ship. A crew member described the blaze as "like trying to put out hell itself."

Murphy's law went into full effect, as everything that could go wrong did. Flammable paint spread the fire, the captain fanned the flames by going into the headwinds, lifeboats were inaccessible, the crew had never practiced a fire drill, safety equipment crumbled in their hands as they tried to deploy it, life jackets failed. Women held tightly to the railings while children clung desperately to their skirts, but once they hit the water, they were helpless. "With sure death from fire behind, the women . . . waited until the flames were upon them, until they felt their flesh blister, before they took the alternative of the river," the *New York Times* reported.

Tragically, there were only 321 survivors out of the approximately 1,350 passengers. Although the water was relatively shallow and the distance to shore wasn't far, so few women knew how to swim, and so many had on clothing that made it difficult to navigate the waters, that what was supposed to be a leisurely day trip turned into a disaster.

The incident aboard the *General Slocum* deeply shook the community, its effects reverberating across the country. In the aftermath, people shifted their perspective to view swimming not only as a sport but also as a public health and safety issue equally vital to either sex. Municipalities nationwide unveiled campaigns that urged women to learn to swim, and cities offered lessons to their residents. It became a mixed-gender activity, which might previously have been a little scandalous, but now, because safety was at stake, it began to become accepted by even those with more-conservative leanings.

As Americans were learning these water lessons, it was also the perfect time for swimsuit reform. A year before the *General Slocum* tragedy, a book was published called *Athletics and Out-door Sports for Women* that encouraged physical activity both as a curative agent and for recreation. Each chapter was written by a different expert; the one on swimming was penned by a gentleman named Edwyn Sandys, who was far from impressed by contemporary women's swimwear. "Judging from the practical and rational point of view, anything more absurd and useless than the skirt of a fashionable bathing-suit would be difficult to find," he wrote. In case you're wondering how a man would know that, he took it upon himself to try on a ladies' suit to experience it firsthand. "Not until then did I rightly understand what a serious matter a few feet of superfluous cloth might become in water," he wrote, reflecting on how he sank nearly instantaneously.

There was an alternative, and Australian Annette Kellermann wore it well. She learned to swim as a way to strengthen her legs after falling victim to rickets, a softening and weakening of bones, in her youth. By age thirteen, she had healed, and by fifteen, she was winning races, on her way to becoming an Australian national champion. She moved to the U.K. and, at age nineteen, attempted to swim the English Channel in 1905. The venture failed, but the long hours she spent in the chilly waters made an impression.

Later that year, Kellermann was invited to give a performance for the royal family at London's Bath Club, but she knew she couldn't wear her typical uniform. Down Under, the style for both men and women was a sleeveless one-piece that stopped mid-thigh. Conventions differed in England (just as they did in the U.S.), calling for women to wear skirted suits. That would interfere with Kellermann's ability to actually swim, so she improvised, sewing a pair of black tights onto her suit to create a sleek one-piece bodysuit. Modern swimwear was officially born.

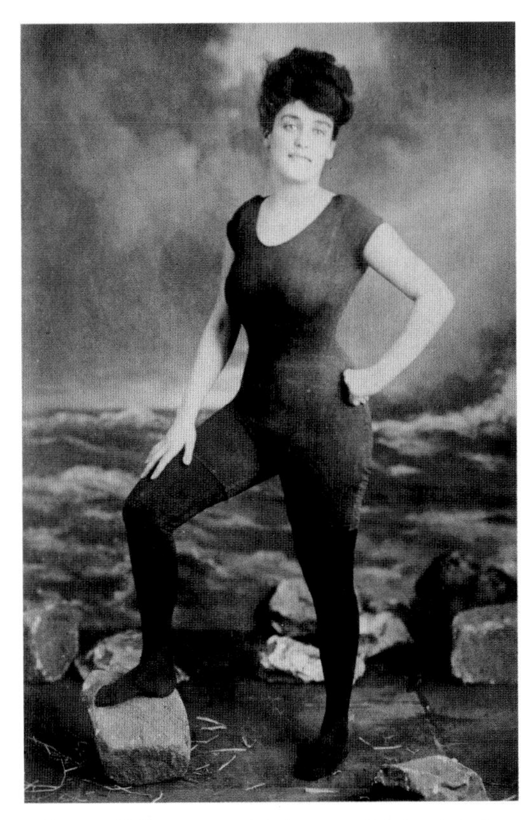

Annette Kellermann models her nonskirted swimsuit, which became highly fashionable.

Dubbed the Kellermann, this newfangled swimsuit was not only fashionable—and, no doubt, a bit titillating in its tightness, even though it covered most of the body—but it was also far more practical than its predecessors. Kellermann talked up her streamlined suit, heralding its lighter weight and enhanced mobility as safety features. "I am certain that there isn't a single reason under the sun why everybody should not [wear] light weight suits," she wrote in 1918. "Any one who persuades you to wear the heavy skirty kind is endangering your life." By the 1920s, multiple manufacturers were making a Kellermann-style swimsuit, widely available in department stores (previous generations of swimmers had to sew their own bathing costumes).

The savvy businesswoman and talented athlete became enormously popular as an entertainer, a silent-film star, and a health and fitness expert. In 1919, she wrote one of the first celebrity exercise books, which encouraged swimming and barbell training, called *Physical Beauty: How to Keep It*. She clarified that her concept of beauty wasn't gorgeous blond hair or a perfect nose but "vitality, health, magnetism, and symmetry."

Kellermann used her fame to encourage women to live active lifestyles—she wanted to remove the barriers that were keeping women weak. Through lectures and articles, she broke down the swimming strokes and gave advice on how to avoid common pitfalls, such as getting a sunburn. (Cold cream slathered on the face was the trick.) She advocated getting rid of restrictive clothing that made one timid. "You cannot be brave," she said in one lecture, "if your diaphragm is squeezed and you can't breathe properly." At these lectures, she sometimes took the shocking step of disrobing, revealing her one-piece suit underneath, in all its loose-on-the-diaphragm glory.

ANNETTE KELLERMANN KNEW SWIMMING HAD the power to save lives and reduce timidity. But she also knew something else about swimming: women were really good at it.

"Women are especially well fitted, mentally and physically, to become proficient in the art of natation," she wrote (using another word for swimming, for those not up on their French-inspired terms). She wasn't wrong. It

“MY LOVE FOR SWIMMING REALLY CAME FROM THIS LOVE OF NOT WEARING MY PROSTHETIC LEGS. I FELT VERY EQUAL IN THE WATER.”

JESSICA LONG

PARALYMPIC SWIMMER

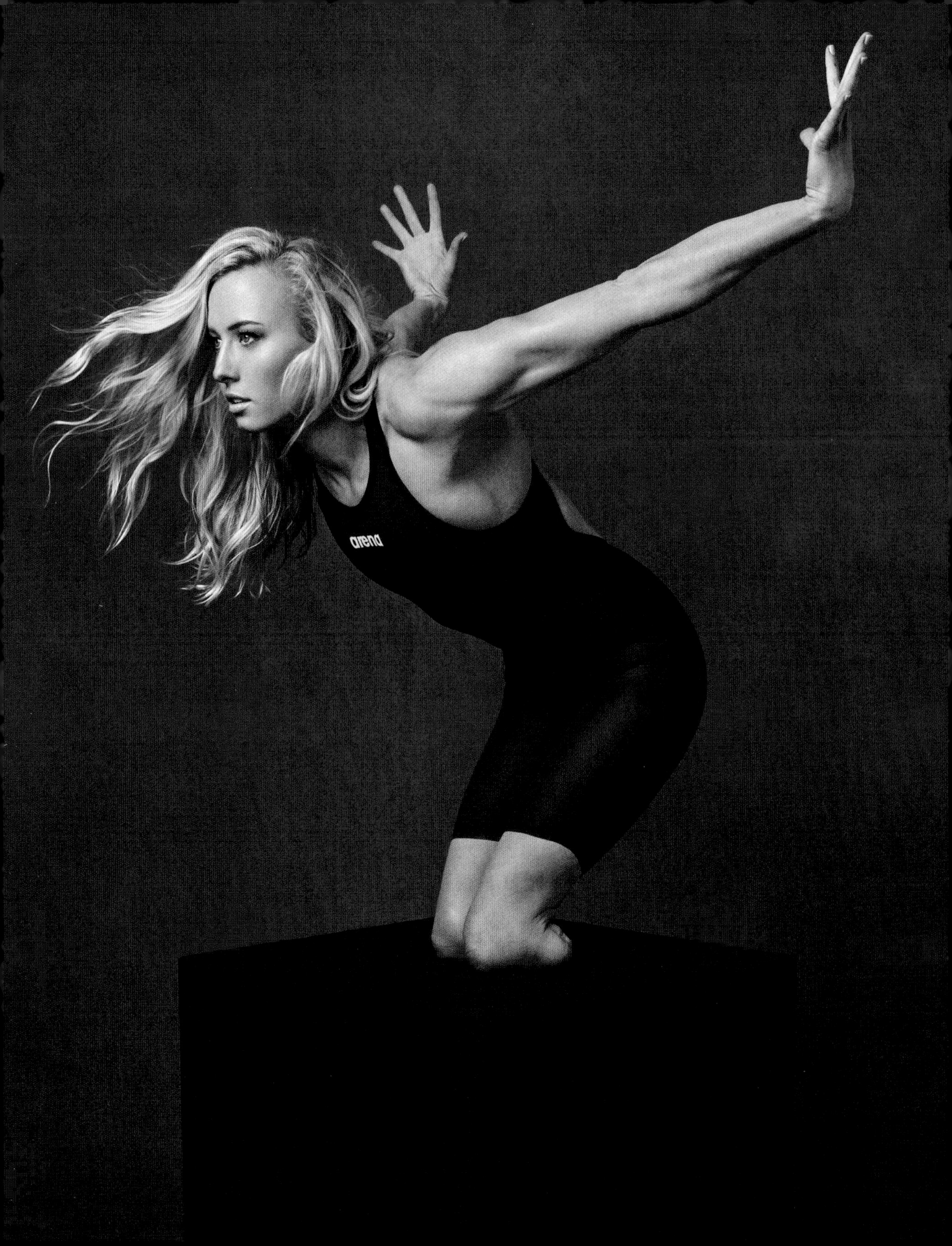
arena

was clear that when given the opportunity to learn to swim, women excelled at covering long distances. In 1910, at the age of fifteen, Rose Pitonof won the eight-mile Boston Light Swim, the only competitor to successfully complete the race. She became a well-known vaudeville performer, staging water demonstrations that dazzled crowds while encouraging spectators to learn lifesaving water skills.

"She was just a teenager taking on these amazing challenges," says modern-day endurance swimmer Jaimie Monahan. "She represented this new kind of freedom and experience just as women were permitted to be swimming."

The opportunity to swim wasn't easy to come by, though. In the beginning of the twentieth century, a woman could actually be arrested for swimming in the ocean without her stockings. (Kellermann herself claimed to have been arrested for indecent exposure while wearing her signature suit in Boston in 1907, after she'd already become popular. "I can't swim wearing more stuff than you hang on a clothesline," she protested.) The machines that towed swimmers out to deep water were outfitted with a "modesty hood" that spared everyone the sight of the female form in a clingy suit. Even as tighter swimwear started popping up everywhere, beaches implemented rules to try to regulate it. While these dress codes applied to everyone, women bore the brunt of the critical attention. Chicago's Clarendon Beach hired a female "beach tailor," who would make alterations on the spot, adding longer skirts or closing up armholes that looked loose.

"The first female swimmers were women on the fringes, women willing to hurl themselves into the water in bathing suits that exposed their flesh," Karen Karbo writes in *Nike Is a Goddess*. "They were brazen, wanton." As such, the pioneering natators were usually eccentric adventurers who lived for an adrenaline rush.

One of the most brazen of all was Gertrude Ederle, who described the sea as "like a person" she'd known a long time. On August 6, 1926, while slathered in a mix of olive oil, lanolin, petroleum jelly, and lard in an effort to stay warm and protected from poisonous jellyfish, the twenty-year-old became the first woman to successfully swim the English Channel from France to England. It was especially remarkable because she had to swim fourteen extra miles due to bad currents during her journey. Two million people greeted her in a ticker-tape parade when she returned home to New York, the biggest parade the city had ever seen. (It was a markedly warmer reception than she had received from a British immigrations officer, who demanded a passport not long after she staggered onto shore.)

Not just the currents were against her. On the exact day Ederle completed the fourteen-hour, thirty-one-minute swim—making her a faster swimmer than any woman *or* man alive—the *Daily News* of London predicted she would fail, publishing an editorial that proclaimed: "Even the most uncompromising champion of the rights and capacities of women must admit that in contests of physical skill, speed and endurance they must remain forever the weaker sex." No word on whether they ran a retraction the next day.

THE OPINION PIECE PROBABLY SEEMED like a safe bet at the time the editors were drafting it, because, as we've seen, years upon years of conventional wisdom said that women just didn't have it in them to do hard things. This kind of "wisdom" had to be pushed against and disproved time and time again.

"For centuries women have been shackled to a perception of themselves as weak and ineffectual," Colette Dowling wrote in 2000's *The Frailty Myth*. "The perception has been nothing less than the emotional and cognitive equivalent of having our whole bodies bound. . . . The frailty myth was driven by men's repressed wish to preserve dominion. To make the myth viable, society constructed elaborate ways of keeping women cut off from their strength; of turning them into physical victims and teaching them that victimhood was all they could aspire to."

Whether intentional or not, society's efforts to keep women from accessing their strength intrudes not only upon their freedom but on their very safety. Consider the right to acquire the self-defense skills of martial arts, the ability to flee a bad situation developed in running, and the flotation lessons learned in swimming—all of these could save you one day. Not to mention the inner strength cultivated through the mastery of a new skill. These are rights to be celebrated and relished, even as it boggles the mind that they were ever withheld. The science of today shows that even the increased muscle mass developed through resistance training is correlated with a longer life. "There's research showing that the amount of muscle and strength you have as you're reaching senescence is a positive predictor of life span from there, so jacked people at sixty live longer than not-jacked people at sixty," says champion powerlifter and coach Greg Nuckols. "It just helps people be more resilient as everything else starts breaking down."

GLOBALLY, MEN ARE STILL MORE likely to know how to swim than women, which holds true even in the U.S., where girls fill more of the ranks of competitive swimmers. In recent tsunamis, such as those in Bangladesh and Indonesia, women died at far higher rates, at least partly attributable to cultural norms around girls learning to swim.

Freedom of movement and being in control of one's body are not privileges, they're fundamental human rights. Strength is perfunctory, not just a luxury, a fact well understood by the swimmers-turned-vaudeville-performers who incorporated lifesaving skills into their acts in the early decades of the 1900s. If it hadn't been for the Annette Kellermanns and Rose Pitonofs and Gertrude Ederles of the world a century ago, we might still not have known that a woman is fully capable of taking a dip in the ocean and emerging invigorated—and, most important, alive.

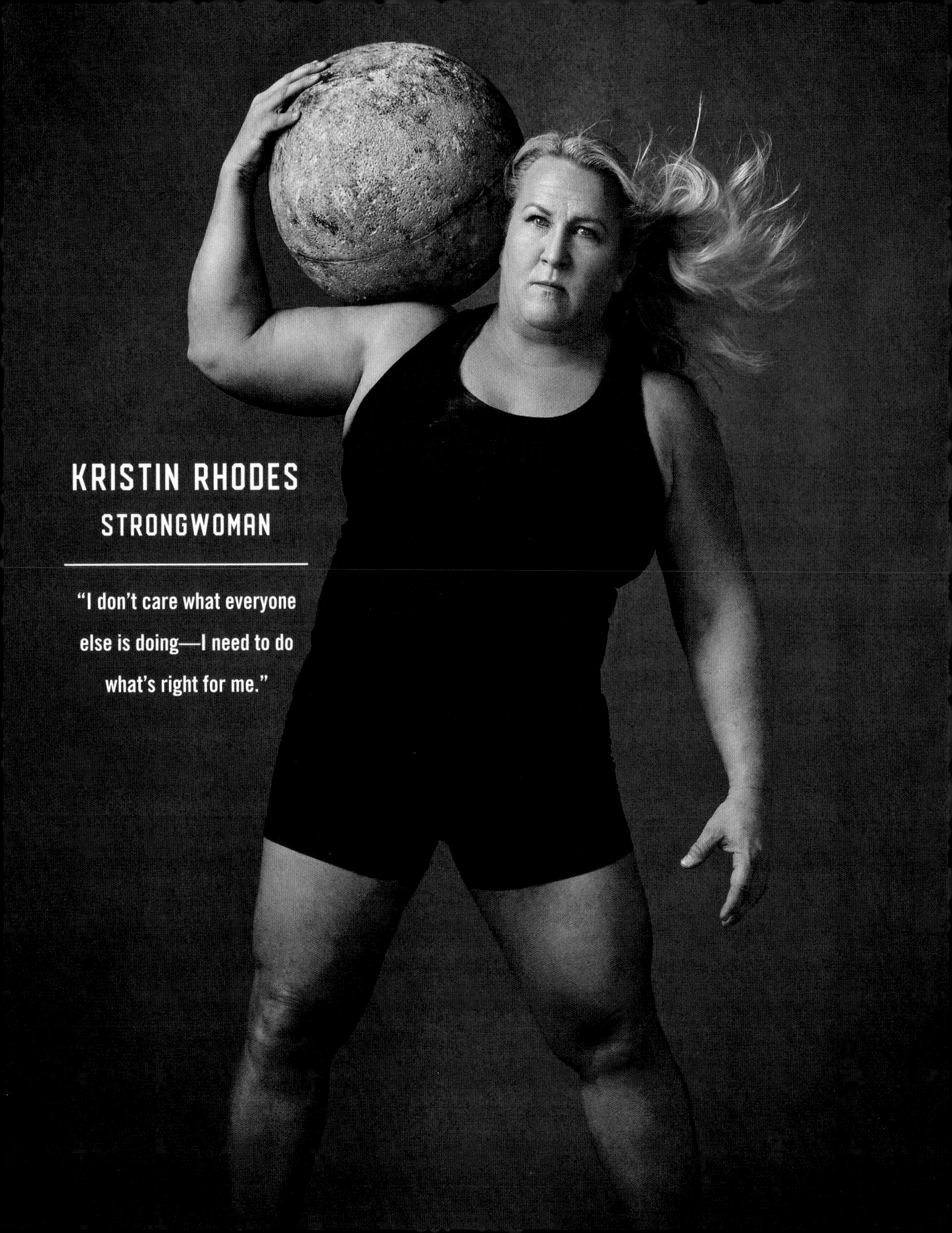

KRISTIN RHODES

STRONGWOMAN

"I don't care what everyone else is doing—I need to do what's right for me."

CHAPTER 4

THE SANDWINA EFFECT:
STRONGWOMEN, THE CIRCUS, AND SUFFRAGE

While circuses have mostly been buried by the sands of time, in the Victorian era, they were a great transmitter of culture. With no Internet, television, or even radio to communicate ideas, information spread much differently from how it does today. When the circus came to town, everyone hit the pause button on regular life to go and watch. They might see exotic animals they'd never laid eyes on before—think tigers, zebras, and giraffes—or people performing tricks that were pushing the bounds of human potential. The circus celebrated what was possible. It was colorful and loud, enveloping the senses in a novel way, with every smell, sight, and sound so far removed from the daily experiences of the attendees that it made an indelible impression. The headliners were today's version of the Hollywood elite. Performing all over the country—and often internationally—they commanded a large and diverse audience, wielding a surprising amount of influence.

Even in this context, some circus stars captivated the public in a way that was an exception to the rule. And if anyone can be described as exceptional, it's Katharina Brumbach.

It all started in the back of a circus wagon in Vienna in 1884, when strongwoman Johanna Nock Brumbach gave birth to her first daughter, Katharina. The proud father, Philippe, stood six feet, six inches tall and supposedly had fingers so big that you could "put a half-dollar through his wedding ring." Combine that stature with Johanna's fifteen-inch biceps, and it's not surprising that young Katie was strong. She could do handstands at age two and started lifting weights in adolescence. By the time she was a teenager, Philippe was offering men who came to see their small circus one hundred German marks to beat her in a wrestling match—but she never lost. (In fact, she won more than just every match in which she was challenged. She also gained a husband in one of the poor guys she defeated, acrobat Max Heymann, who said he fell in love with her while he was lying on the floor, fresh from his trouncing.)

A mix of undeniable strength, show(wo)manship, and a pleasing visage thrust her into the spotlight. She made a name for herself, quite literally, in New York in 1902, when she went toe-to-toe in a lifting throwdown with an audience member who just happened to be the most famous bodybuilder in the world at the time. Widely considered to have the perfect proportions, Eugen Sandow once wrestled a muzzled lion for kicks and had abs that appeared to be chiseled from marble. When Katie floated 300 pounds over her head and he could only get the weight to his chest, the crowd was in disbelief. Sandow was, too. (Or so the story goes. Circus performers were notorious for embellishing a detail here and there, but we do know that Katie could outlift most men.)

Katie began calling herself Sandwina—a feminine version of Sandow—and rode the wave of admiration that came from her impressive stunts. She later scored a starring role in Barnum & Bailey's Greatest Show on Earth, earning a good living at a time when most women in this line of work were relegated to sideshow acts or tossed around as props. When discussing vaudeville acts of the era, the authors of *Venus with Biceps*—a pictorial look at strongwomen through history—write that a woman "was something to lift, throw, or project through the air, an ornament in tights, but seldom the star of the show."

Not so for Sandwina, who could hardly be described as anyone's prop. Rumor even had it that Siegmund Breitbart, dubbed the "Strongest Man in the World" in the 1920s, preferred not to appear in cities at the same time that Sandwina was scheduled to perform. Although he could lift baby elephants and pull wagons with his teeth, he wanted to avoid being upstaged by the "Lady Hercules," as she was affectionately known.

The Lady Hercules · Katie Sandwina
A Combination of female Strength, Form & Beauty.

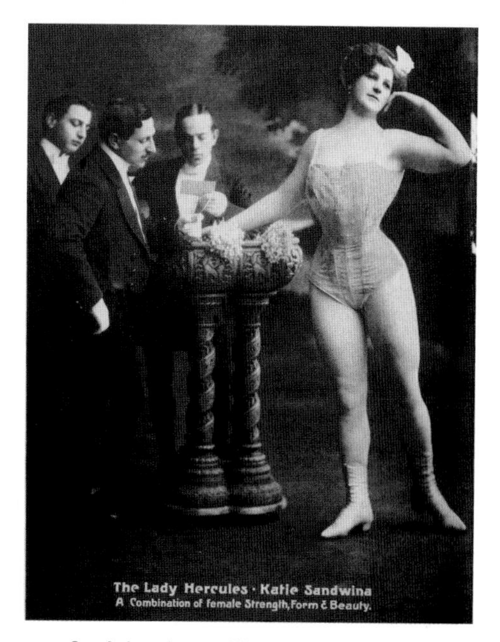

Sandwina shows off her lauded figure in a promotional photo.

Sandwina was a woman of many talents. She broke chains, juggled cannonballs, lay on a bed of nails, and lifted three men at a time. When she raised her husband above her head, she didn't appear to struggle at all; it looked more like "a little light housework with a feather duster," influential journalist Kate Carew observed. The night before she gave birth to her first son, she performed in two shows. (He grew to weigh 50 pounds by the age of two and liked to run around with a 25-pound dumbbell as a toy, a far cry from the wooden blocks his contemporaries busied themselves with.) Sandwina didn't lose a step as she got older. One writer who saw her perform in his youth gushed that at the age of forty-six, she was still capable of breaking a Bulldog chain, the kind farmers used to tether bulls and oxen, designed to withstand a pull of 8,000 pounds. She was, in all ways possible, as strong as an ox.

THE WAY SANDWINA WAS SOLD to the public illustrates how strength was still something of a threat to femininity unless packaged in a certain way. At an event meant to drum up publicity for the circus, a dozen doctors examined Sandwina and declared her the perfect specimen—all 210 pounds of her. (She was quite tall, somewhere between five-nine and six-one, though accounts vary.) After the doctors sized her up, the *New York World* wrote: "The feminine Hercules has a wonderful figure, full of symmetry and not marred by a display of muscles."

Although Sandwina's frame might be considered bigger than desirable by mainstream standards today, a grand stature, a sturdy build, and a robust constitution were the components of one of several beauty ideals in the early 1900s. While big muscles weren't part of that package, Sandwina's didn't seem obtrusive, which was evident to anyone who saw her in evening attire.

"Her arms, which can raise 240 pounds above her head, are supple and smooth enough to project from a ball gown," journalist Carew wrote in 1911. "No horrid lumps of muscle, dears—just a little ripple under the skin, like mice playing in a mattress."

St. Louis Post-Dispatch reporter Marguerite Martyn used another animal analogy when she called the strongwoman "panther-like," exalting her "attributes of swiftness and grace and the faculty of concealing great strength within soft, subtle curves.

"As she swings gracefully into the arena on supple, slender, silk-encased limbs, your vision seems to dilate a bit, your eyes adjust themselves to magnified but perfect womanly proportions," Martyn wrote, "and she is more like a new and shining statue of an heroic Venus than the antique and gnarled god of strength."

Sandwina's strength was sort of like a hidden talent. She appeared like any fresh-faced, full-figured woman of the era yet was capable of mind-boggling feats. She was performing Superman-like skills while looking like Clark Kent. If she'd sported hard, rippling muscles instead of "mice playing in a mattress," she would have lost that everywoman exterior reporters found so fascinating. All the adulation for Sandwina was in the context of how her strength wasn't at odds with her femininity but well within the confines of it. The two *could* coexist—if one had the right look. And Sandwina did.

The circus promoters were shrewd. They knew if they wanted to gain broad appeal for a female strongwoman, they would need to play up the idea that she was beautiful, not brawny. They had just the right person to present in this fashion, because by all accounts, Sandwina had a striking face and a graceful way of moving. Additionally, it didn't hurt that she was married. She was often asked to talk about her kids and her domestic pursuits—she cheerfully cooked and did the laundry—and magazines printed her parenting advice. (Suffice to say the list of things she fed her children would increase your grocery bill by an amount you might find untenable.) All of this reminded everyone that while she was an outlier, she was still playing by society's rules of what a woman should be, with appealing curves and a strong maternal instinct.

HOW DID CIRCUS STARS GET to be the kinds of public figures whose grocery lists were detailed in newspapers? Having a massive, entertainment-hungry audience wherever they roamed helped. "The circus was a totalizing nomadic city," says Janet M. Davis, author of *The Circus Age: Culture & Society under the American Big Top*. "Literally the whole town would shut down as people came to the show."

At these events, spectators had an opportunity to see women playing roles that looked very different from what they experienced and observed in everyday life. Organizers such as P. T. Barnum (who had learned as a museum proprietor that appealing to women and children was a smart thing to do) reinforced the ideal of a lady as modest, respectable, and well mannered by marketing to that sensibility, but the circus also presented alternative images of an alluring woman. "Within the show grounds, you had this spectacle of women defying those very stereotypes of Victorian frailty; these muscular bodies were doing things indistinguishably from male circus performers in terms of their strength and their agility and their ability to tumble," Davis says. "In that sense, what's going on actually in the ring or the sideshow is a place where those norms were being very much defied, so you've got a rhetorical confirmation of Victorian ideals about gender, but in practice, you have this total pushback."

As the more liberated New Woman archetype took hold—a feminist ideal from the 1890s through the 1920s of a woman who stood for education, independence, sexual autonomy, marriage based in equality, and social change—circuses included women as ringmistresses and clowns, traditionally male roles. If you wanted to see a woman who didn't conform to the prevailing norms, you could step right up to the circus and see some big gender barriers broken down under the big top.

EVEN WITHIN THE UNCONVENTIONAL WORLD of the circus, Sandwina was not your typical circus performer. For one thing, she was well paid, up to $1,500 a week. Careers for other female performers might not be as lucrative, but there were other women who made a name for themselves—and often a fierce name, at that. There was Athleta, who could waltz with three men on her shoulders. One of her signature tricks was getting in a crab position with a seesaw on her abs of steel, a horse balanced on each end.

Then there was Vulcana, the beautiful daughter of an Irish minister, who as a teenager once stopped a runaway horse in the middle of a street in England and freed a wagon whose wheels had locked up. Articles about her accomplishments illustrate how she, too, defied gender norms while simultaneously reinforcing them. "When you hear or read of a woman of this description, you naturally conjure up visions of a large, heavy, mannish-looking person, devoid of the soft feminine graces which must ever enfold the type of true womanhood," an article in *Sandow's Magazine of Physical Culture* said. "But you have only to see Vulcana to realise that there is nothing masculine about her, in spite of her strength."

There was also Minerva, who could lift 700 pounds from the floor, one-hand press

100 pounds overhead, and, standing in a ten-quart bucket, hoist a 300-pound barrel of lime to her shoulders without disturbing the bucket at all, demonstrating tremendous balance to accompany the strength. She once lifted eighteen men at a resort near Washington, D.C., and she had a surefire system for fueling herself for that kind of stunt.

"Eating is about the principal part of my existence, and I always have the best I can possibly procure," she told a reporter. "For breakfast I generally have beef, cooked rare; oatmeal, French-fry potatoes, sliced tomatoes with onions and two cups of coffee. At dinner I have French soup, plenty of vegetables, squabs and game. When supper comes, I am always ready for it, and I then have soup, porterhouse steak, three fried eggs, two different kinds of salads and tea. For every meal I have a bottle of the best wine I can procure."

AS POWERFUL AND WELL FED as these one-named women were, there was one thing they lacked, at least early in their careers: the right to vote.

The circus was like a fun-house mirror for the dynamics within general society. As women grew restless with their lot in life, the circus stars who embodied an image of strength gained even more acclaim. "By the late nineteenth century, as women became increasingly involved in public activism, the fight for suffrage, marital property reform, and public education, one of the things you really see as a striking change is women become the focal point of circus advertising campaigns," historian Davis says.

Some of the women wanted to use that star power for greater good. Popular equestrian performers such as Josie DeMott Robinson, May Wirth, and Victoria Davenport were outspoken in their support of suffrage. They were mocked by reporters (as most suffragists were), but they were a natural fit to advocate for the cause. "There is no class of women who show better that they have a right to vote than the circus women, who twice a day prove that they have the courage and endurance of men," said suffragist Elizabeth Cook.

A common argument against women at the ballot boxes was that voting should be reserved for those who possessed the physical strength to defend that right, if pressed in war. Naturally, that was intended to mean men only. When reporter Martyn met Sandwina, she saw firsthand the folly in this line of thinking.

"If physical strength is to decide supremacy in this government of ours, why then here was Sandwina displaying more strength than the average man, be he voter or otherwise," Martyn wrote. "Wouldn't it be a good idea to nominate the young Amazon leader of the suffrage movement and follow her to victory?"

In 1912, Sandwina became vice president of Barnum & Bailey's eight-hundred-member suffrage group, earning her the nickname "Sandwina the Suffragette." Some believe this may have been yet another ploy for circus publicity, but the strength and independence she embodied were undeniable.

"The anti-suffragists who go to the Barnum & Bailey Circus at Madison Square Garden, and see Sandwina, the German strong woman, lift her husband and two-year-old son with one arm, tremble for the future of the anti-cause," a 1911 article in the *American* said. "When all women are able to rule their homes by such simple and primitive methods they will get the vote—or take it."

THE CIRCUS WAS A NATURAL home for the suffrage movement. Here were women making their own money, traveling the world, and sharing the same spotlight as men, which gave them a unique perspective.

"You earn salaries," horseback rider Robinson told her fellow performers in 1912. "Some of you have property. You have a right to say what shall be done with it. You want to establish clearly in the mind of your husband that you are his equal. You are not above him, but his equal. You are not slaves." (Upon hearing this, a circus man barged into the meeting and removed his wife and daughter, calling Robinson's ideas "nonsense" and saying he was hungry for dinner.)

For most women, running away to join the circus wasn't part of their master plan.

But many realized they did deserve some say in the trajectory of their lives and that their voices were just as important as a dinner-loving man's. And ultimately, it wasn't a crazy circus implement like a 600-pound cannon or a razor-thin high wire that helped convince them but a more accessible piece of equipment: the humble bicycle.

Prior to the late 1880s, bicycles were considered death-defying contraptions that only young daredevils would dream of attempting to ride. That was for good reason; even the names of the early models imply danger. Consider the boneshaker, which offered an extremely bumpy ride on wooden wheels, or the penny-farthing, whose seat was up to five feet off the ground, putting riders at great risk for hard falls. (In fact, you had to know how to properly "take a header" to ride one—that is, land safely after catapulting headfirst over your handlebars.)

The safety bicycle changed everything. The wheels were approximately the same size; the pneumatic tires provided a smooth ride, even on paved roads; and functional pedals made turning corners simple.

It was the 1890s version of going viral. In 1897 alone, 2 million were sold in the U.S. But the bike was more than just a fitness craze—it changed the very landscape of women's rights.

OF THE ESTIMATED 2 MILLION American women who rode bikes in the 1890s, the president of the Women's Christian Temperance Union, Frances Willard, was a particularly prominent one. Until her sixteenth birthday, she'd run wild on the frontier of the Wisconsin Territory, gardening and plowing her own little field. Then, like nearly all other girls, she was bound in long skirts, corsets, high heels, and pinned hair for adulthood. "In my heart of hearts," she said of the conventional norms, "I felt their unwisdom even more than their injustice." She later recalled: "I remember writing in my journal, in the first heartbreak of a young human colt taken from its pleasant pasture, 'Altogether, I recognize that my occupation is gone.'"

More than thirty years went by, and while she certainly stayed busy—particularly in her role with the WCTU, which campaigned for labor laws, prison reform, and suffrage—something was missing. Even with all her activism, all her petitioning, preaching, and publishing, she realized that her mental and physical life were out of balance.

Maybe it wasn't practical to return to her "beloved and breezy outdoor world" of romping out in nature, felling saplings with an ax rigged up from old iron, but there was something she could do.

So in 1892, at the age of fifty-three, Willard learned to ride a bike.

It took her three months of practicing fifteen minutes a day to conquer the machine she called Gladys, so named because learning to ride made her glad. It wasn't a big time commitment, she pointed out, only thirteen hundred minutes, or twenty-two hours, or "less than a single day as the almanac reckons time."

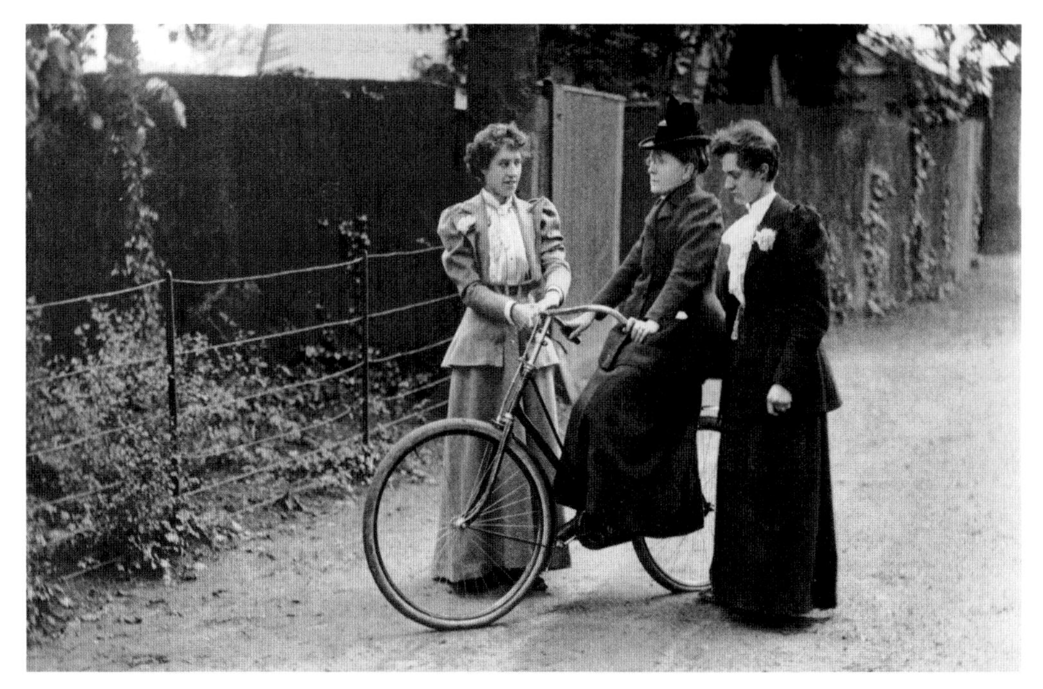

Frances Willard learns to ride a bicycle with the help of friends, circa 1894.

The freedom and unbridled joy of her younger years came rushing back, and she hoped that as a public figure, she would inspire other women to draft behind her.

Willard understood as well as anyone that cycling really meant more than fresh air and a little exercise—it meant independence. "I began to feel that myself plus the bicycle equaled myself plus the world, upon whose spinning wheel we must all learn to ride," she wrote. "She who succeeds in gaining the mastery of such an animal as Gladys, will gain the mastery of life."

THE BICYCLE WAS NOW NOT just a ubiquitous transportation device; it became a symbol of suffrage. "To men, rich and poor, the bicycle is an unmixed blessing, but to women it is deliverance, revolution, salvation," wrote Anna de Koven in *Cosmopolitan* magazine's August 1895 issue (under the name Mrs. Reginald de Koven). "It is well nigh impossible to overestimate the potentialities of this exercise in the curing of the common and characteristic ills of womankind, both physical and mental, or to calculate the far-reaching effects of its influence in the matters of dress and social reform."

Many physicians were supportive of this new hobby, saying that it helped ease childbirth by developing the uterine muscles. They also cited the positive effects that riding in the fresh air had on exhaustion and depression.

Notably, cycling changed the way women dressed. Fashion may seem trivial, but clothes mattered. Shoving that corset into the back of a dresser drawer let loose a lot more than just a woman's internal organs. There was now a very good reason to wear more-sensible garments. Baggy knee-length trousers known as knickerbockers, bloomers, and higher hemlines all came into vogue.

"If women ride they must, when riding, dress more rationally than they have been wont to do. If they do this many prejudices as to what they may be allowed to wear will melt away," Willard wrote. "A woman with [bustle] bands hanging on her hips, and dress snug about the waist and chokingly tight at the throat, with heavily trimmed skirts dragging down the back and numerous folds heating the lower part of the spine, and with tight shoes, ought to be in agony."

The prejudices did begin to melt away, although the thawing process took some time. While women were invigorated by the freedom that the bike brought—they could actually go somewhere on their own, without a chaperone—they still had to contend with the naysayers who argued that the saddle on a bike would induce the start of menstruation or cause contracted vaginas and collapsed uteruses or become a secret way to masturbate. Some even suggested that bicyclists invited lewd commentary from less-than-gentlemanly passersby by showing their ankles.

If none of that deterred them, opponents could warn women to avoid "bicycle face," an unseemly condition in which the eyes bulged and the jaw clenched, forever.

"I think the most vicious thing I ever saw in all my life is a woman on a bicycle," wrote a contributor to the *Sunday Herald* in 1891. "I had thought that cigarette smoking was the worst thing a woman could do, but I have changed my mind."

Filling your lungs with a carcinogenic substance doesn't practically change the power dynamics in society, but learning that you can control where you go and when you go there sure does.

In the fight for suffrage, bikes sometimes played a direct role. Campaigners used them to travel to spread their message and hung banners off the handlebars, and in at least one instance in England, suffragists blocked Winston Churchill's motorcade with their bicycles to make a point. There was more to it than that, though. Getting that little taste of freedom was the spark that lit the fire to pursue more rights.

It's no coincidence that as the New Woman ideal emerged, she was often portrayed on a bicycle.

THIS WASN'T THE FIRST TIME an athletic display was tied to suffrage. Back in the early pedestrianism days, America's first female star of the sport, Bertha von Hillern, squared off against fellow competitor Mary Marshall in a series of six-day races. (Von Hillern was so popular in the 1870s that you could buy a "von Hillern hat" and her photo in department stores. She was called "an apostle of muscular religion" by one paper.) Around the same time, the Supreme Court barred women from arguing cases in front of it. The editor of the *New York Times* drew a connection between the two. "Though women may not practice in the Supreme Court, they may walk for money," he wrote.

"Obviously those who have aspirations above baby-tending, dishwashing, and writing for the magazines, will refuse to accept walking matches in lieu of possible forensic honors. Let such be encouraged, however, by what has been accomplished. The world moves—is moving. To-day it is the walking match; next it will be the coveted entrance to the Bar. After that, who shall tell how soon the ballot will come."

THE NINETEENTH AMENDMENT, GRANTING WOMEN the right to vote, officially went into effect in 1920. Sandwina the Suffragette played her small (or perhaps not so small) part in making that happen.

She brought women's physical capabilities into the public eye, at a time when women were just beginning to learn what fitness could do for them, that swinging an Indian club could make their bodies feel more alive or learning to ride a bicycle could provide a sense of accomplishment. She showed them what was possible—or if not exactly possible, at least an ideal they could strive for.

Journalist Carew might have been Sandwina's biggest fan, and she had many. "In her presence you can think of nothing small—only of large things, like nature, motherhood, and creation," she wrote. "She is as majestic as the Sphinx, as pretty as a valentine, as sentimental as a German schoolgirl, and as wholesome as a great big slice of bread and butter."

And after 1920, as powerful as a person with the right to vote.

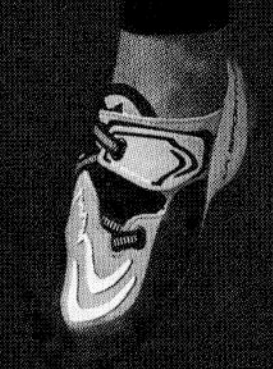

MARGO HAYES

CLIMBER

“Climbing is a social activity, where we work together and support one another. When we have a partner at the other end of the rope, our life is in their hands.”

CHAPTER 5

BEACH BABES:
PUDGY STOCKTON AND THE CROWD-PLEASING LADIES OF MUSCLE BEACH

By the time the final years of the Roaring '20s rolled in like an ocean wave, women were registering to vote in record numbers and becoming increasingly active in politics on both a local and a national scale. Dress codes loosened, waistlines dropped, and hemlines rose. Employment options were somewhat limited to a handful of occupations, but women's independence was growing. Little did they know that in a decade's time, there would be more job opportunity than ever before—although not for a reason anyone would have wanted.

But before men shipped off to fight in World War II and Rosie the Riveter's "We can do it!" message galvanized women into physical work in factories and shipyards to fill the void left by soldiers, the world was plunged into the Great Depression.

With little left, people had to hold on to each other, and one very fit group of people took that adage quite literally.

• • •

LIKE ANY OTHER U.S. CITY in the early 1930s, Santa Monica was struggling, and there would be no reprieve for the Southern California community when an earthquake ravaged the landscape in 1933, reducing many buildings such as homes and schools to piles of rubble. Physical education instructor Kate Giroux came up with an idea to restore some normalcy: have the city erect a central playground until the schools could be rebuilt.

It seemed a small gesture, but anything that could buoy spirits at this time was worth a shot. So with money from the Works Progress Administration, a Depression-era program that employed people for public works projects, Santa Monica turned Giroux's vision into a reality.

Yet it wasn't only the children who benefited. The playground at Mussel Beach, so called because of the abundance of shellfish, began attracting gymnasts and acrobats who needed a soft place to land (literally and figuratively) as they practiced their routines while waiting for the vaudeville shows to begin hiring again after the economic downturn.

With equipment such as bars and rings, Mussel Beach gained a reputation, enough to attract the type of beachgoer who made the punny name change inevitable. (At least, as one story goes, though no one seems to agree on the original name.) Weightlifting demonstrations, hand-balancing feats, gymnastics and acrobatic displays, adagio performances, and bodybuilding competitions kept the participants in shape and passersby entertained.

As time went on, crowds flocked to watch the activities, and the city of Santa Monica added a gymnastics platform, ping-pong tables, volleyball nets, and more. Snack shops lining the beach sold ten-cent hamburgers and five-cent ice cream cones. Jukeboxes blasted music from the pier. Working out was far from a priority for the majority of people at the time, but this turned out to be just the distraction they needed. A few heckled, but most appreciated the energetic displays of athleticism.

“Those who didn’t understand what we were doing called us ‘Muscleheads,’ ” wrote Harold Zinkin, the first Mr. California and inventor of the Universal Gym Machine, in his book *Remembering Muscle Beach*. “Although the term stung at the time, history has proven that we were on the right track, and that ‘muscle’ isn’t a dirty word.”

Zinkin wasn’t the only one who went on to fame and fortune. Many future fitness scions got their start at Muscle Beach, including Vic Tanny, the father of the health club; Joe Gold, an early bodybuilder and founder of Gold’s Gym; and Jack LaLanne, the godfather of fitness himself, who inspired people to put down the sugar and pick up the dumbbells (and buy a lot of juicers). On a per-square-foot basis, more fitness legends got their start on the sands of Muscle Beach than anywhere else in the world. Trace the origins of the modern health movement, and all roads lead to this Pacific Ocean enclave.

While plenty of notable men buzzed around the beachfront property, doing flips and tricks and pressing big loads overhead, it was a woman who rose to the top of the human pyramid.

THE QUEEN OF MUSCLE BEACH was born Abby Eville in 1917. After graduating from high school, she landed a sedentary job as a telephone operator. In a situation similar to that of many office workers today, she didn’t like the way she felt as a result of sitting all day. Although she’d always been petite, for once, she was starting to live up to the “Pudgy” nickname her dad had given her in her youth.

In the 1930s, the owner of York Barbell and founder of *Strength and Health* magazine, Bob Hoffman, was trying to get a message across: lifting weights would not make a woman look manly. But the idea wasn’t catching on. The only people who paid him any attention were those already converted. The general public didn’t buy that weight training was an appropriate activity for ladies.

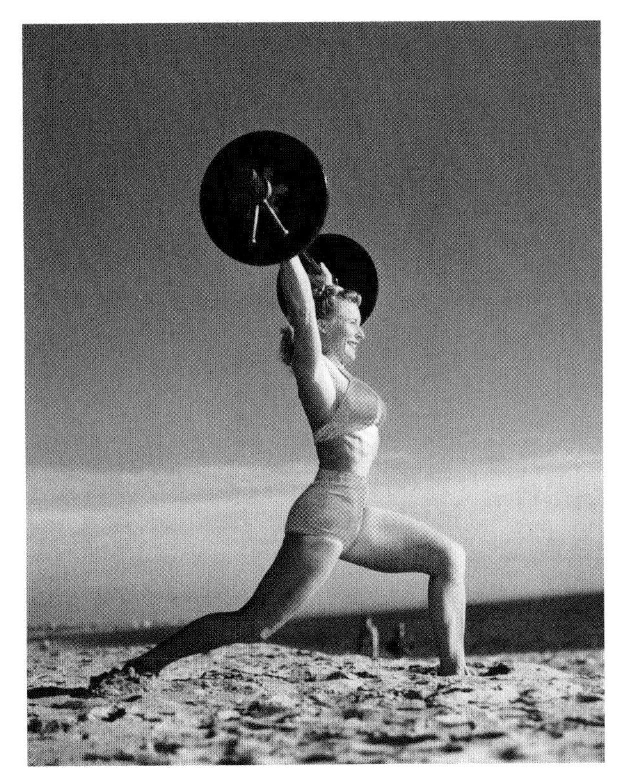

Pudgy Stockton performs a 100-pound split jerk on the beach in Southern California.

Enter Pudgy. Her boyfriend (and later husband), UCLA student Les Stockton, hooked her up with a set of dumbbells and a York training course. She was reluctant at first; she wanted to "reduce," in the parlance of the time, not add bulk. But when she tried to find advice on what would help her accomplish her goals, she discovered that scant information existed for women wanting to work out, so she decided to trust Les and see where it took her. At the beach, Pudgy started by learning to do a handstand, which she would later describe as the main turning point in her life. She quickly found that she loved acrobatics and had a talent for it. She began spending her afternoons off from her split shift at the telephone company practicing tricks at Muscle Beach.

Practice indeed makes perfect. Before too long, Pudgy could hoist an oversize dumbbell into the air or hold a handstanding man above her head. She could push a barbell from her chest with a guy carefully balanced on top of it. She could balance on someone's hands while pressing 100 pounds above her head, or she could reverse the trick and be the one supporting the barbell presser.

Soon she was making public appearances doing acrobatic tricks alongside a few men, and by the fall of 1939, she appeared at the halftime show of a

UCLA-versus-USC football game, introduced as "Pudgy and her boys." At just under five-foot-two and 115 pounds, Pudgy had a sex appeal and a softness that endeared her to a wide audience—muscularity wasn't so threatening when it came in a wholesome package. By the end of the 1940s, she'd appeared on the covers of more than forty magazines and within the pages of countless others, catching the eyes of photographers for both fitness titles and mainstream publications such as *Life*.

She wasn't the first weightlifting woman who captured the public's attention, nor was she even the first to be celebrated for her good looks. But she differed from someone like Sandwina, whom journalist Kate Carew described as a "gigantic and beautiful young creature." At five-foot-ten-ish and 200-plus pounds, Sandwina had measurements that weren't likely for the average woman (who also probably didn't dream of lying on a bed of nails with a 200-pound anvil on her stomach, spectacular as that might have been to watch).

Pudgy was different in that she was so much more average. She was strong, yes, but in a very girl-next-door way. Her dad didn't have fingers that were the size of a half dollar, and her mom didn't have biceps that were bigger than most men's. The typical woman could more easily see herself in Pudgy's shoes, frolicking on the beach under warm rays of sunshine. Pudgy's chin-length hair was coiffed just right, her smile always warm and engaging. Vibrant, pretty, and strong—suddenly, that was something women very much wanted to be.

AS WORLD WAR II CONSUMED the country in the 1940s, men left for battle, women's roles were changing, and Pudgy was just the kind of girl who represented the new normal. "Petite Pudgy Stockton with her glowing skin, shining hair, miraculous curves and amazing strength appeared on the golden sands of Muscle Beach and became emblematic of the new type of woman America needed to win the War," writes Jan Todd, a scholar of strength sports.

In July 1944, Pudgy began writing a column for women called "Barbelles" in *Strength and Health* magazine, then the most influential fitness magazine around. She wrote about noteworthy women like Muscle Beach comrade Edna Rivers, shown deadlifting 505 pounds with ease, but she also celebrated the everywoman. She featured Kay Brougham of Montreal, who was in a car accident that left her with fifteen broken ribs, a collapsed lung, and a dislocated knee. The mother of six worked her way back to health by taking up weight training, pressing a 14-pound dumbbell above her head for fifteen reps on each side. "Her achievements and the stamina required to overcome the effects of a bad accident are to be highly praised and admired," Pudgy wrote. "If a person with such a handicap can attain such fine results, it is certainly conclusive proof that those of us who are enjoying good health and the full use of all our appendages can make even faster gains."

The tone in her column was always kind and inspirational, and it was the same in her many letters to fans, who wrote with questions or to express thanks. She gave a lot of practical advice, such as recommending bowling shoes for lifting (the best option at the time) and a two-piece bathing suit for ease of movement (stretchy leggings were not yet a thing, so her mom improvised in creating Pudgy's workout wear). She also wisely encouraged readers to take it slowly, starting with light weights before working their way up. She made sure they knew real progress would take some commitment. "It will mean sacrifice to the extent that you will have to [forgo] some free time that would otherwise be spent on dissipating pleasures," she wrote. (Even though that great dissipating pleasure of Netflix didn't exist yet, people nonetheless found ways to distract themselves.)

Pudgy stressed that lifting weights was for everyone—young and old, single and married, with children and without—and she took everyone's achievements seriously. Accompanying one particularly sweet photo from 1944, she wrote this caption: "Maureen O'Brien, age 3 1/2, has been following a regular training program with fine results. She is pressing 5 pounds."

Weightlifting had previously been associated with grunting, grimacing men, but Pudgy appeared joyful as she worked, her face radiating with accomplishment. As appealing as she made lifting look, there were always naysayers who felt weights really weren't appropriate for women. One reader wrote in: "Many women gave me queer looks at the mere mention of it as though it were on a par with rum running or bank robbing!"

Lifting weights may not have been illegal the way smuggling alcohol was, but it did provide a dose of adrenaline that women were realizing they liked, and Pudgy's encouragement helped others feel confident that they were making a good choice. In times that tried the nation and the world economically and emotionally, her upbeat voice was a ray of hope.

IT WASN'T JUST WOMEN WHO benefited from Pudgy's motivation. Heavyweight weightlifter Jim Bradford, who won silver medals in two Olympic Games and four World Championships, gave Pudgy her due in his strength journey. "Man, let me tell you—that Pudgy Stockton was a carrot on the stick for many a guy who's taken up the weights," he said, "if they were man enough to admit it, that is."

One anonymous veteran who landed in a Los Angeles area hospital after World War II was definitely man enough to give Pudgy props. "One afternoon I wandered down to Muscle Beach and saw a little blonde with the most beautiful muscles I had ever seen," he said. "I knew it had to be Pudgy Stockton. Right then and there I took 'stock' of myself. I'd let myself become a mess—and the damn War hadn't helped. I went home, joined the Y, and started working out. It was that simple." She wasn't the first fit person he'd laid eyes on, but she was the one who left the biggest impression. "I had seen most of the Mr. Americas up to that time, and I've seen many since," he continued. "But that one woman, that one afternoon of my life, helped me change my life around, even though nothing else ever had. Because of her, I'm a different man."

PUDGY WAS ARGUABLY THE MOST prominent female face of Muscle Beach, but she wasn't alone. The Muscle Beach Weightlifting Club had more than one thousand members, about twenty of whom were women. The percentage may have been tiny, yet, like Pudgy, this group was small but mighty.

The very first woman to garner attention on the beach for her dazzling displays of strength and grace was Relna Brewer McRae. At just over five feet tall, she looked a lot like Pudgy: conventionally pretty, petite, blond, with a well-proportioned body.

She didn't start as a superstar. She made her way to the beach as a fourteen-year-old by tagging along with her brother, who thought it would do her health some good. McRae had been burned by boiling water in an accident when she was eleven, and as a result, her right shoulder was four inches lower than the left. To recover, she began by simply hanging from a bar, stretching her scar tissue until it hurt.

That helped her rehab her shoulder to the point where she could stand up straight. From there, McRae progressed to swinging around a high bar, then to somersaulting off the rings. Soon she was called the strongest girl in the world and backed up the title by bending iron bars and walking on wires.

McRae relished the attention, and she collected quite a colorful array of fun facts to share at parties: she could tear a Los Angeles phone book apart with her bare hands, she served as a decoy for Marilyn Monroe to help her slip away from the paparazzi, and a photo of her supporting three other women—one on her shoulders and one standing on each of her thighs—made the rounds to at least fifty major newspapers.

As she and Pudgy lifted weights one day, she remembers a man yelling out, "Fake, fake. You can't tell me that weighs anything."

She invited to him to come up and give it a try. Sure enough, when he attempted to lift her 135-pound, very real barbell, he found himself unable to get it to budge—and probably regretting his heckling. Circuses and vaudeville shows sometimes used sleight of hand to stage tricks, but the women's strength at Muscle Beach was no illusion.

YOUNGSTERS, TOO, HAD THEIR SPOT on the sand. As a ten-year-old, Pat Keller McCormick started spending her free time at Muscle Beach, where a gym owner introduced her to barbells. She got super strong, to the point where she could do thirty-five handstand press-ups in a row, more than any of the men on the beach.

McCormick was also a daredevil, the kind who'd do cannonballs off bridges to splash boats as they went past. She put that talent to good use as an adult by winning diving's coveted double-double: gold medals in both springboard and platform diving at back-to-back Olympic Games in 1952 and '56. She remains the only woman ever to have done so.

"At age 10, I remember participating in adagio and athletics at Muscle Beach," she later said. "I attribute my body strength, for which I became known in diving, to that part of my life. At Muscle Beach, I was constantly lifting men up off the ground. Because weight training was not a part of our normal training regimen in my era, I was fortunate to have those activities at Muscle Beach."

ON MAPS FROM THE 1940S, "Muscle Beach" appears in a bigger font than "Santa Monica," yet by the end of the 1950s, it was gone, at least officially. (Another,

“THERE ARE YOUNG WOMEN OUT THERE WHO FEEL LIKE I REPRESENT SOMETHING THAT GIVES THEM HOPE. IT BRINGS ME GREAT JOY THAT I CAN BE AN EXAMPLE FOR YOUNG DANCERS WHO ARE FOLLOWING THEIR DREAMS.”

STELLA ABRERA

BALLET DANCER

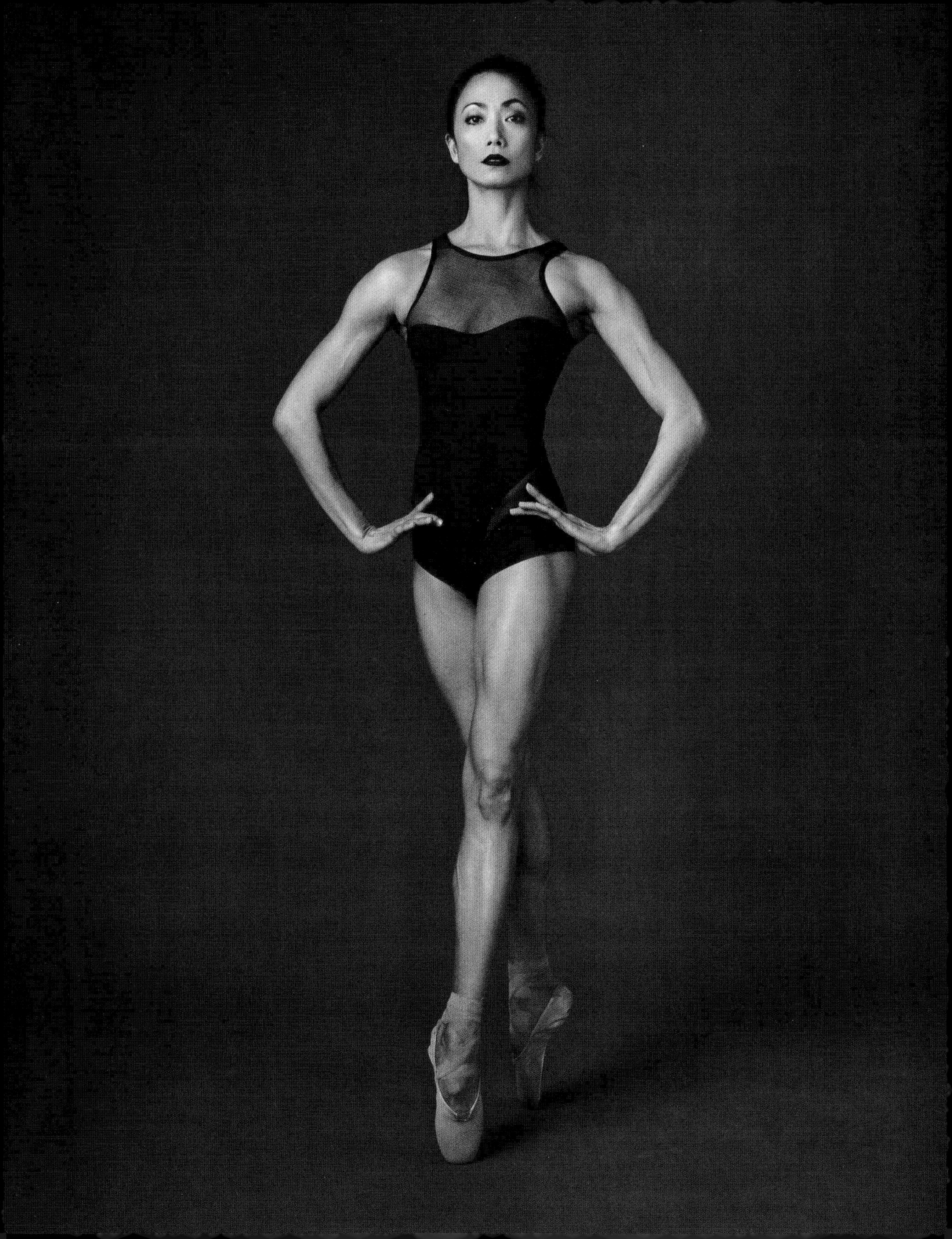

more bro-tastic version later sprang up in nearby Venice.) For a brief moment in history, the right people at the right time turned it into the phenomenon it was. "What might have felt like fun and looked like entertainment was the beginning of a fitness education for an uninformed nation," Zinkin wrote in 1999. "As the war stressed our minds and our bodies, that nation took a long, serious look at fitness. . . . Before long, what we believed and practiced at Muscle Beach started sounding less and less crazy."

Instead of keeping their secrets close to the chest, as some athletes do for competitive reasons, members of the community all shared tips with one another. They freely traded information on fueling their bodies with salads and raw milk before others paid attention to nutrition, subscribing to the notion that a rising tide lifts all boats. "Every time you came down, it was fun because you made new friends, you learned to do new things," Pudgy said. "It's hard to describe what a wonderful place it was."

If ever there were an original #fitfam, this was it. "I remember this camaraderie, this group of friends—they'd meet there every weekend," says Randy Boelsems. His mom, Paula Unger Boelsems, was a fixture at the beach, known for her graceful postures in flight. "Everywhere you went, somebody was doing a handstand, a backbend, a cartwheel."

They all took turns spotting one another and developed the kind of bond that's helpful when you're precariously balancing on the shoulders of someone who's standing on the outstretched abdomen of a guy doing a backbend. Many remained friends for their entire lives. "The girls, flying through the air, had to hold their position [and] completely trust their catcher. The spotters, who would prevent the fall of participants in risky positions, must be completely trustworthy, and they were," wrote Les Stockton, recalling that no one ever suffered a serious injury.

“The most important thing we had at Muscle Beach was the friendships,” Joe Gold said.

That kind of unerring faith in one another was inspiring, in a way that resonated deeply in an era when faith was often tested. There was an equality on the beach, an idea that anyone who wanted to learn was worthy of teaching. Men, women, boys, girls—if you were willing to put in the work, you could join the family.

THIS WAS FITNESS FOR A greater good. The regulars showed that working out wasn’t just a job, although many of them became successful in business because of their physical strength. It was a lifestyle, not just for the genetically gifted or privileged but for anyone and everyone at the level that made sense for them, even three-and-a-half-year-olds pressing five pounds.

It looked easy, though it wasn’t. It also looked fun, and it was. But mostly, it was hard work—Armand Tanny, brother to Vic and a winner of both Mr. America and Mr. USA, called the relentless training “the grief grind” because of the tireless effort put into perfecting stunts and strengthening muscles.

And perhaps no one on the beach worked harder than Pudgy Stockton. She hosted the first sanctioned weightlifting competition for women in 1947, wrote her “Barbelles” column for a decade, and opened a cozy women’s-only health club with wallpapered walls and benches that looked more like furnishings than utilitarian implements. Her reach went far beyond the crowds that gathered around a platform next to the Pacific Ocean.

“Every woman bodybuilder who puts on a swimsuit and steps up on the posing dais, every woman weightlifter who strains under a clean and jerk, and every woman powerlifter who fights through the pull of a heavy deadlift owes a debt of gratitude to Abbye ‘Pudgy’ Stockton, who helped make these modern sports possible," writes Todd, who in 2009 was the first woman inducted into the International Powerlifting Hall of Fame. (Pudgy, by the way, changed the spelling of her first name from Abby to Abbye after marrying Les.)

When Pudgy first picked up those dumbbells, she couldn't have predicted what would result. All she understood at the time was that sitting at a desk for eight hours a day wasn't benefiting her body. "I know when I first started, it gave me a feeling of being able to do something that not a lot of people could do," she said. "I had so much more confidence in my outlook on life and about myself."

To his credit, Les recognized the special qualities that Pudge—his name for her—possessed, and he considered it a privilege to be her husband. "In the 40's era of male macho and men divorcing women because they couldn't handle the spouse making more money than they did, [I] was not one of these," Les wrote. "When Pudge began receiving international recognition for her exploits and herself, I enjoyed every moment of it. Did I resent being billed as 'Pudgy Stockton and Her Husband,' 'Mr. & Mrs. Pudgy Stockton'—not even once!"

LES AND PUDGY, RELNA AND Pat, and all the athletes of Muscle Beach brought it to life. It appeared effortless for these legends, tanned and chiseled, to perform superhuman feats. They were gifted, no doubt, but what they really represented was not raw talent as much as hope. During the Depression and World War II, that was in short supply. People wanted to believe that if they just kept going, things would get better. Sure, the Muscle Beach denizens' above-average flexibility, strength, and creativity were inspiring. But it was also the dream that a better day was around the corner that these athletes exemplified as they lifted one another up, in all ways possible.

They showed up every day, whether or not anyone was watching, and slowly mastered skills. They made daily choices in regard to training and nutrition that made incremental differences. They delighted in moving their bodies, even when their bodies didn't want to move. In the end, they showed that over time, anything is possible and that strength breeds resilience. Maybe you couldn't solve all the world's problems, but you could wake up just a little bit stronger than you were yesterday.

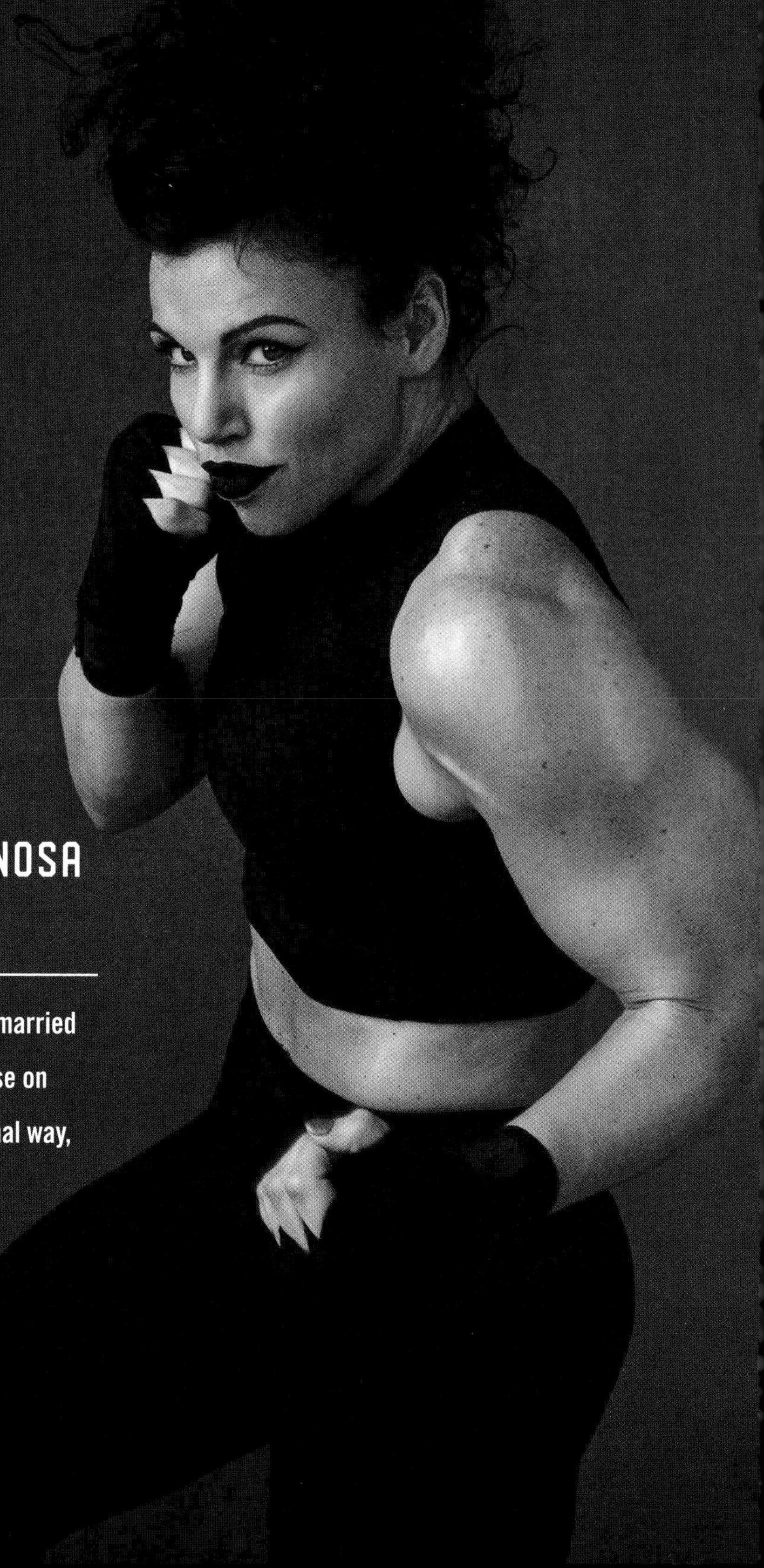

ALICIA NAPOLEON-ESPINOSA

BOXER

"If it was up to my family, I'd be a nurse married with five kids living in a two-story house on Long Island. I'm not doing it the traditional way, I'm doing it my way."

CHAPTER 6

UNLADYLIKE:

WHEN A BABE IS NOT CONSIDERED A BABE

Hope probably should have been in short supply for a young Mildred Ella Didrikson, even in the days before the Great Depression took the country under its shadowy grip.

Babe, as she was better known, grew up in Beaumont, Texas, in the 1910s and '20s, the sixth of seven children born to poor Norwegian immigrants. To help the family, she sewed gunnysacks for a penny apiece. She was a bit of an unruly child, known for running around barefoot, always caked in mud. Her neighbors thought her rude and loud, not a popular combo for a little girl. Babe found the hobbies for little girls, such as hopscotch and jacks, plain old boring. She preferred to be on the sandlot with the boys, ripping off home runs. She also wasn't much of a student, forced to repeat a grade before eventually dropping out.

But when Babe looked in the mirror, there was no hopelessness there. She didn't see the dirt or grime or poverty. She saw an athlete.

BABE WASN'T JUST ANY ATHLETE. She was like a hybrid of Michael Jordan, Katie Ledecky, Tiger Woods, Jackie Joyner-Kersee, and a really good bowler all rolled into one package. In a 1955 issue of *Sports Illustrated* that posed the question "Is Babe Didrikson the greatest all-around athlete of all time?" her biggest competition among respondents was the legendary Jim Thorpe, who played football, basketball, and baseball, along with winning Olympic gold medals in the pentathlon and decathlon. (Of course, there had to be a little sexism in the responses—as the chief of French Army Engineers said, "A woman the greatest athlete? You Americans are so droll.")

Most professional athletes tend to excel at one sport, maybe two. But the muscular Babe excelled at nearly everything she tried—and on a staggering level. Just consider this abbreviated résumé:

- Track and field: Two gold medals and a silver, plus two women's world records, in the 1932 Olympic Games (in 80-meter hurdles, javelin, and high jump).
- Golf: Ten major championships and thirty-one tournament wins in the Ladies Professional Golf Association (LPGA).
- Basketball: All-American three years in a row.
- Baseball: World record for the longest throw by a woman.
- Miscellaneous: Accomplished in diving, roller-skating, bowling, tennis, swimming, boxing, volleyball, handball, billiards, and cycling.

Was there anything she didn't play? "Yeah, dolls," she once said.

IN 1932, THE AMATEUR ATHLETIC UNION held a national meet to determine who would get the slots for track and field in that year's Olympics. Sports clubs from all over the country sent their most talented lineups. Babe showed up alone, as a one-woman team.

Her coach knew it would garner publicity—but he also knew she was more than capable of putting the other teams to shame. Babe astonishingly won the entire track meet, racking up 30 points as she competed in eight of ten events that day, frantically running from one to another, and winning six outright. The second-place team, which fielded twenty-two athletes, managed only 22 points.

After collecting a trio of medals a couple of weeks later at the Los Angeles Olympics—Babe remains the only female ever to win Olympic individual medals in running, jumping, *and* throwing—she was a bona fide star. But female athletes didn't have a ton of moneymaking opportunities in sports at the time, so in 1933, she joined the vaudeville circuit, where she earned up to $1,200 a week, a life-changing sum in an age when women could expect about six cents an hour for difficult work. Her act involved hitting plastic golf balls into the audience, running on a treadmill, playing the harmonica, and cracking some well-timed jokes. It went remarkably well, but she longed to be a competitor again. This time, she set her sights on a new game to master: golf.

DEFINING ONESELF SOLELY AS AN athlete, as Babe did, was an unusual thing for a woman to do. Sandwina and Pudgy were athletes, too, but they were also well-rounded wives and mothers—and beautiful ones, at that. Babe, described by one writer as "a hard-bitten, hawk-nosed, thin-mouthed little hoyden from Texas," had a sharp and angular face that made her the target of particularly cruel criticism and none of the soft curves that tended to make muscularity more culturally acceptable on a woman.

Reporters were also suspicious because she seemed indifferent to men. It had been a long time since an independent woman like that had catapulted herself into the spotlight for her sporting achievements, maybe not since the Greek huntress Atalanta chafed at settling down with a suitor.

"It would be much better if she and her ilk stayed at home, got themselves prettied up and waited for the phone to ring," wrote Joe Williams in the *New York World-Telegram*.

For the most part, Babe let these kinds of comments rush by as quickly as her fastball pitch—which once struck out Joe DiMaggio—but she *was* bothered by the idea that she was too masculine, that she immersed herself in sports because she couldn't catch a man. The truth was that she immersed herself in sports because she was a competitor at heart, and the rest didn't much matter.

THE KIND OF SINGULAR FOCUS Babe had on winning could be admirable in men, but it felt misplaced in a woman. She just didn't seem like a lady. Ladies wore bras and girdles, even if that constricted their movement. Ladies put on makeup and did their hair. Ladies were polite and demure. Unlike her contemporary Pudgy Stockton, who always had a kind word of encouragement for other women, Babe preferred trash-talking before a competition. She was known to walk into a locker room and ask her opponents who was playing for second. We can argue about whether that was *sportsmanlike*, but instead, the conversation was always around whether she was *ladylike*.

Throughout history, women have largely been expected to fulfill two very important roles: wife and mother. From these two roles stemmed a cascade of other expectations: a woman should be pretty (in order to attract a man and have children), straight (in order to marry a man and have children), and docile (in order to keep a man and have children).

Being strong simply didn't contribute to any of those traits. In fact, some believed it actively detracted from them. It's hard to look pretty when you're sweating, your face contorted with effort. And when you're facing down an opponent or yanking around a barbell, you can't be docile and expect to be successful.

But the real anxiety was often related to something far less superficial than looks or temperament. Many worried that to be a strong woman meant being *into* women. That was the undercurrent of concern when reporters wondered about Babe's dating life, and in fact, she did live with a female companion in the final years of her life.

The nature of their relationship is debated, and Babe never acknowledged it as a romantic one in public. Even if it had been, that's no surprise. When tennis superstar Billie Jean King was outed decades later, in 1981, she lost an estimated $2 million in endorsements overnight. By the mid-1990s, attitudes had evolved, but 46 percent of women athletes said in a survey that their involvement in sports caused others to assume they were lesbians. More than half of female coaches and sports administrators said the same.

These underlying assumptions hurt sporting women of all sexual orientations. Retired U.S. soccer star Abby Wambach, who is gay, has spoken out on not wanting to reinforce "the cliché that exists in women's sports, that it's a lesbian world, because that's just not how it is." Whether accused of being something you're not or blamed for being something you are, neither is productive in encouraging females to play sports, especially adolescent girls. The Women's Sports Foundation says that discrimination based on real or perceived sexual orientation and gender identity is an issue that students still face. "Girls in sports may experience bullying, social isolation, negative performance evaluations, or the loss of their starting position," the organization says. "During socially fragile adolescence, the fear of being tagged 'gay' is strong enough to push many girls out of the game."

While the stereotype persists in some circles that sports and sexual orientation are somehow related, this faulty logic doesn't deter nearly as many girls from getting strong as it did even a generation ago. It helps that attitudes toward those who don't identify as cisgender and/or straight have become more accepting. That said, it would be a mistake to think the idea that "really good female athlete equals gay" isn't still a thing. Look no further than the reaction to WNBA star Brittney Griner telling reporters she was gay a few days after being drafted as the number one pick in 2013. Hardly anyone cared. Or, more accurately, hardly anyone was surprised. Yet when NBA player Jason Collins made a similar announcement shortly after, the sports world erupted.

"Call it the double standard of sports sexuality: Male athletes can't be gay, but females are assumed to be," explained New York University professor Jonathan Zimmerman. "Far from shocking our sensibilities, Brittney Griner's announcement confirmed them."

This cultural bias puts the onus on female athletes to prove that they're straight, to show off their femininity. Women who are gay are not nearly as likely to be playing sports as stereotypes might have you believe. While 68 percent of high school seniors play at least one sport, only 21 percent of LGBTQ high school seniors do. To get maximum participation, sports should be more inclusive in general, unmoored from any assumptions about sexual orientation.

"Across our society, the taboo on male homosexuality remains far greater than the one on lesbianism. That makes it more difficult for male athletes to come out as gay, but it also extends the historic burden on sportswomen to prove they're not," Zimmerman wrote. "And it makes it harder for all of us to be what we should be: ourselves."

THE SPORTS JOURNALISM TIDES FINALLY turned in favor of Babe in 1938, when she married George Zaharias, a professional wrestler she met during a golf tournament in which she was the only woman competing.

Life magazine ran the headline "Babe Is a Lady Now: The World's Most Amazing Athlete Has Learned to Wear Nylons and Cook for Her Huge Husband." Nylons and cooking—she really hit the big time!

Marriage also apparently transformed her body, giving her bigger breasts, a smaller waist, and thirty-seven-inch hips, according to one creative writer, who noted that she was previously rumored to be a boy. (Perhaps it didn't hurt that Zaharias was tall and strong at six feet tall and 225 pounds, and next to him, Babe looked small.) While it's possible that wardrobe tweaks and filling out a bit with age might have affected Babe's appearance, the ring on her finger didn't materially change her measurements, only the way she was perceived.

Even Paul Gallico, once the highest-paid sportswriter in the country, was impressed. And he wasn't exactly a champion of female athletes. "No matter how good they are they can never be good enough, quite, to matter," he wrote. (One exception was female swimmers, otherwise known as "handsome young girls in revealing bathing-suits.")

Although he had previously called Babe an ugly duckling with a hatchet face and said she was so good at what she did "because she would not or could not compete with women at their own and best game—man-snatching," he changed his tune once she was perceived to have been domesticated. According to Gallico, Babe became a "splendid woman" who made the "transition from the man-girl who hated sissies to a feminine woman." (It's worth noting that Gallico lost a golf match and a footrace to Babe six years before she got married, which didn't seem to bring out his kindest words.)

Babe's impressive career was dismissed by Gallico and others as a passing fad, a detour into tomboyishness while she was on her way to her true destiny as a lovely lady. As one reporter put it, "Along came a great big he-man and the Babe forgot all her man-hating chatter."

While marriage was certainly not Babe's most interesting accomplishment, you wouldn't know that from the breathless proclamations of sportswriters after she tied the knot. That simple act of saying "I do" proved that she could be tamed.

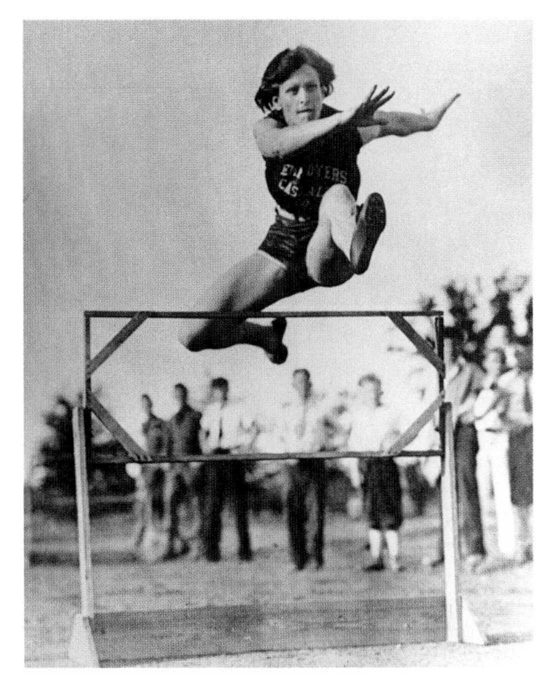

Babe Didrikson clears a hurdle at a track meet in 1932.

Unmarried women are dangerous. Wild. Unpredictable. Unable to be controlled.

So when a woman like Babe got married, the critics could all breathe a sigh of relief. She might still bound over hurdles faster than the average man—Babe's athletic career continued after her wedding, all the way until her untimely death from colon cancer at age forty-five—but that was trivial stuff. To someone of a certain mindset, she proved that when it really mattered, she would fall in line with the feminine ideal, the storybook narrative that always ends in happily-ever-after marriage to a fairy-tale prince.

THE THIRD PIECE OF TRUE ladyhood—as common convention dictated, at least—was motherhood. Babe never had children, and in her day, people thought muscular women were doomed to a life of infertility with all that activity. Pudgy Stockton, who came of age at the same time, heard all the arguments about fitness and family being incompatible. "People used to say that if women worked out, they would become masculine-looking or wouldn't be able to get pregnant," she told *Sports Illustrated Women*. "We just laughed because we knew they were wrong."

For those who didn't understand the benefits of athletic training, Victorian-era logic still lingered, with many convinced that the uterus would shift and loosen with exercise, rendering it an unfit womb. Some believed that women's muscles were slack compared with the taut ones found on men, and trying to strengthen them would only change the fibers in a way that was detrimental to childbirth. Too much exertion was a recipe for exhausting your body beyond its limitations, and conventional wisdom said that wasn't something you could expect to bounce back from.

We have lots of counterexamples today of high-performing athletes who have become moms, including beach volleyball player Kerri Walsh Jennings capturing the gold while five weeks pregnant in London in 2012, heptathlete Jessica Ennis-Hill winning a silver medal at the 2016 Olympics after having a son, and ultramarathoner Sophie Power breastfeeding her three-month-old during the middle of a 106-mile race in 2018. Still, kids undoubtedly complicate the trajectory of an athletic career.

"Maybe having a baby on the tennis tour is the most rebellious thing I could ever do," Serena Williams told *Vogue* after having her daughter, Olympia. (She chose that name, by the way, after googling names that derive from words for "strong.")

Kikkan Randall, who along with teammate Jessie Diggins won the United States' first-ever Olympic medal for the women's cross-country skiing team, was generating buzz well before the historic win at the 2018 Winter Olympics. That's because out of the 109 female athletes from the U.S., Randall was the only mom. (On Team USA, 20 of the 135 male athletes—14.8 percent—were fathers.)

Randall, who had her son in 2016, put a lot of effort into getting back into shape. She worked out twice a day during pregnancy and returned to hiking and biking within a month of delivery, but there were still issues she didn't anticipate. When Randall tweaked some back muscles just getting out of a chair, she discovered that while her aerobic capacity and muscular structure remained solid, her inner core muscles weren't what they used to be.

"In some ways, I was pleasantly surprised at how much I could do, but in other ways, it did take a bigger toll on my body than I would've guessed," she told HuffPost. "It did take some patience and diligence to work back."

Most mothers can relate to this on some level, Olympians or not. My mom friends at the gym laugh when they see jumping rope programmed in a workout—bladder control just isn't what it used to be after giving birth.

IN 1928, FOUR YEARS BEFORE Babe won her Olympic medals, the Games debuted the 800-meter distance for women. (For reference, 800 meters is a half mile, twice around a track, and can be run in less than two minutes by the world's best.) Of the eleven competitors, five dropped out before finishing, and five collapsed at the finish line, reported the *New York Evening Post*. It was "not a very edifying spectacle," according to Notre Dame football coach Knute Rockne, who was acting as a reporter at the Amsterdam Games. "The half-mile race for ladies was a terrible event," he wrote. "If running the half mile for women is an athletic event, then they ought to include a six-day dancing contest between couples. One is as ridiculous as the other." The *New York Times* solemnly proclaimed: "This distance makes too great a call on feminine strength." After that, track distances of more than 200 meters were eliminated for women so as to preserve their child-bearing abilities, their frailty, and even their dignity.

It wasn't just men who doubted the ability of women "distance" runners. Even fellow track and field competitor Betty Robinson, an American teen, spoke out against this comparatively longer distance of 800 meters. This was the same young woman who went down in the record books as the first female athletics medalist in Olympic Games history after her 1928 win in the 100 meters. "I believe that the 220-yard dash is long enough for any girl to run," said Robinson, sixteen at the time. "Any distance beyond that taxes the strength of a girl, even though some of them might be built 'like an ox,' as they sometimes say." She admitted that she wasn't a medical expert but said common sense told you that women weren't cut out to run very far. "Imagine girls falling down before they hit the finish line or collapsing when the race is over!" she said. "The laws of nature never provided a girl with the physical equipment to withstand the grueling pace of such a grind."

There's just one problem with the account of the 800-meter race that found women flopping all over the place like fish tossed out of an aquarium: it could use a little fact-checking. Based on footage and photos from the event, it's clear that there were nine competitors, not eleven, and none dropped out before the race ended. The performances were admirable, and the world record was even set that night by a capable runner from Germany, who finished seven seconds faster than any woman had before. In fact, six competitors beat the previous world record. If anyone collapsed in exhaustion, well, that's what can happen when you run your hardest.

Case in point: when the men ran the 800 meters in the 1904 Olympics, long before women would get the chance, two participants reportedly collapsed afterward. One had to be carried off the field. There were no calls to ban them from competing nor accusations that their "physical equipment" didn't pass muster. For men, the event has appeared on the Olympics program without interruption since 1896.

Including the women's 800 meters was controversial from the outset, and it was viewed through that skeptical lens. For the mostly male media establishment, seeing women looking obviously tired was disturbing—exhaustion was not considered beautiful. (Even with this noted bias, it's unclear why so many grossly exaggerated reports came out of the event, but one particularly critical journalist went on to become a writer of sports fiction, so perhaps he was just practicing for his future career.)

BEING CALLED UNATTRACTIVE OR DEEMED infertile was one thing, but when that brash sportswriter Gallico really wanted to stick it to Babe Didrikson Zaharias, he wrote an article in *Vanity Fair* that accused her of being neither female nor male.

In 1933, this was the quickest way to denigrate a female athlete's accomplishments, and questioning one's sex was used on others before and since. During the 1936 Olympics in Berlin, rumors spread that American sprinter Helen Stephens, the six-foot-tall winner of the 100 meters, was actually male. "The accusations followed the logic that no one that tall, with a stride that long, nearly six feet, with a form so graceless, could be anything other than a man," writes Roseanne Montillo in *Fire on the Track*, a book about the earliest competitive female sprinters. In a horrifying turn of events, Stephens had to submit to a genital inspection to clear her name and keep her medal.

It didn't stop there. After Stephens's identity was called into question, the president of the American Olympic Committee, Avery Brundage, said that he believed every female competitor at the Games should undergo a medical test to certify her womanhood. It wasn't a surprising suggestion from a man who didn't hide his disdain for a certain type of athlete. "You know, the ancient Greeks kept women out of their athletic games," he said. "They wouldn't even let them on the sidelines. I'm not so sure but what they were right." (Pat Keller McCormick, the spunky diver who honed her strength on Muscle Beach, wasn't a fan. She snuck into Brundage's room, grabbed a pair of his underwear, and ran them up a flagpole during the 1952 Games in Helsinki.)

IF THAT KIND OF TREATMENT seems like a relic of the 1930s, consider Caster Semenya. Since 2009, the talented middle-distance runner from South Africa has found herself at the center of a controversy about how people are split into categories for athletic competition.

As much as humans like things to fit into discrete boxes, gender and sex are much more complicated. Semenya has a condition called hyperandrogenism, which gives her higher levels of male sex hormones than you would find in the average female; specifically, her testosterone levels are about three times higher.

This all came to light after Semenya won the 800 meters at the world championships as a teenager. The whispers started. Her arms were so big. Her voice was so deep. Her hips were so slender.

She was subjected to an invasive, confidential test that really wasn't confidential at all, as the results were leaked to the press and soon became known worldwide. Instead of a womb, she has internal testes due to a rare chromosomal abnormality.

In May 2019, the Court of Arbitration for Sport ruled that any woman with high testosterone levels who runs a distance of 400 to 1600 meters must enter as a man or take drugs to suppress her hormone production. While the court acknowledged that putting limits on naturally occurring testosterone was indeed discriminatory, it said the policy was a "necessary, reasonable, and proportionate means" of achieving the goal of preserving competition for women. Two days later, before the ruling went into effect, Semenya set a meet record in Doha, Qatar, and won her thirtieth-straight 800-meter race. She was emphatic that she would not be changing her body to suit the court's standards but insisted she would find a way to continue running.

"I think [sport] is all about loving one another. It's not about discriminating against people," Semenya said in 2016. "When you walk out of your apartment, you think about performing; you do not think about how your opponent looks."

If only that were universally true.

THERE HAVE BEEN A VARIETY of ways women have been "proved" to be women throughout sports history. From the 1940s until the 1960s, a certificate from a doctor would usually do. Then it was a physical test (which might morph into a gynecological exam). After that was criticized, the International Olympic Committee turned to various kinds of genetic testing, beginning in 1968.

The testing grew out of a fear that men might be masquerading as women, the very opposite of what the ancient Greeks worried about when they made everyone disrobe before entering the Olympics. The number of times that has occurred in competition is pretty close to zero. An oft-cited example is Dora Ratjen, a woman who placed fourth in the high jump at the 1936 Berlin Olympics, but the story has become tangled over time. One tale goes that a few years after the competition, Ratjen was found working as a (male) waiter and confessed that he'd been forced by the Nazis to pretend to be a girl for three years—a task he allegedly called "most dull"—so that they could prevent a Jewish girl from competing and possibly winning a medal. In reality, Ratjen was born with ambiguous genitalia and was raised as a girl but grew up to feel more like a boy. Ratjen changed his name to Heinrich, stopped competing in athletics, and lived the rest of his life as a man. There's no good evidence that he competed fraudulently or was recruited by the Nazis in an act of deception, as perfect a Hollywood screenplay as that might be.

Not surprisingly, hordes of male hucksters were not caught trying to pull a fast one. Instead, concern that a boy just might pretend to be a girl, despite how low those odds really are, has led to some downright distressing situations. In 1990, a nine-year-old soccer goalie in Texas was asked to pull her pants down at halftime to prove she was a girl. A couple of dads on the other team didn't think a female player could be so good. Her coach refused to let such an inspection take place (because he was a rational human being), and afterward, one of the skeptical dads told the goalie, "Nice game, boy." Fortunately, the talented player took the parents in stride. "I think they should go somewhere and check and see if they have anything between their ears," she said.

In 2011, the system of verifying female athletes became refined. The standard at the time had been a blood test—they looked for a Y chromosome, which triggers male development. But because of the growing awareness that humans don't always develop to be the gender predicted by their genes, they switched to a hyperandrogenism test. If it came back with levels higher than expected, a comprehensive follow-up exam would occur. Women who produced more testosterone than was deemed acceptable would need to medically suppress it.

"In other words, they tried to make the testing of an athlete's femininity something more akin to testing her for doping," *Slate* reported. "The message that came with a negative result shifted from, *Sorry, we don't think that you're really a woman* to more like, *Sorry, you have too much of this performance-enhancing substance circulating in your veins.*"

This seemed better, more objective, to a lot of people, but there were still issues that resulted in these new regulations being suspended. Both men and women produce testosterone. If a man naturally produced more testosterone than the average man, would he be banned from his sport for being "too manly" unless he underwent hormone therapy to reduce his levels? No, no such mechanism is in place for that. And men with genetic anomalies such as XXY chromosomes are not banned from competition.

Semenya's extra testosterone probably does give her an advantage, although how much of one is still something scientists are debating. Michael Phelps's flipperlike feet also give him a major advantage when he's swimming the butterfly. LeBron James's six-foot, eight-inch height makes it much easier for him to dunk a basketball. Archer Brady Ellison has 20/10 vision, which means he can stand twice as far from a target as someone else and still see just as well.

Genetic advantages are, and always will be, part of sports. There are lots of women who have advantages, too, such as the right height for gymnastics, bodies that make better use of lactic acid to power through sprints, or a wingspan perfectly suited to the b-ball court.

While gangly limbs might not be the most desired trait out there, they don't directly oppose femininity the way a muscular figure does. Perhaps that's why we celebrate all these other genetic advantages while trying to tightly control the women who just don't seem like "real" women. So much attention is paid to defining womanhood and deciding how athletic is too athletic, and where to draw those lines falls mostly to men. Accusing a woman of not really being a woman is often a way to detract from her talents, to try to make her feel ashamed and inconsequential, as critics attempted to do with Babe. Through sex testing, we're ostensibly leveling the playing field, but viewed through the eyes of athletes like Semenya, we're instead leveling the bodies of females.

ONCE BABE MARRIED AND STARTED dressing up a little more, she didn't have to worry about the womanhood question any longer. She was heralded as a success story, a tomboy with mud-caked feet transformed into a graceful golfer who wore pearls.

This could have been a natural transition, but Babe's biographers tend to believe she was a woman worn down by society's expectations. It could be that she carefully cultivated her image, portraying her marriage as happier than it truly was and convincing others that she liked makeup more than she really did. Perhaps later in life, she toned down her authentic personality because it was easier that way. The feistiness never fully abated, though. Until her final days, she was making jabs at fellow competitors and focused on winning above all else. Babe was known to make prank phone calls to the other players the night before a tournament, posing as a German woman or a small child, anything to get an edge. When the other women on the golf tour approached her in 1953 about the fact that she was taking appearance fees under the table that no one else received, she set them straight. "Let me tell you girls something," she said. "You know when there's a star, like in show business, the star has her name in lights on the marquee, right? And the star gets the money because the people come to see the star, right? Well, *I'm* the star and all of you are in the chorus. *I* get the money. And if it weren't for me, half of our tournaments wouldn't be." No one argued with her.

Despite a more refined public-facing exterior, at her core, she was still that same cocky young girl who jumped over hedges and played football with the boys, with no regard for how pretty her hair looked.

Coverage of Babe often focused on her supposed shortcomings. Sportswriter Grantland Rice, though, recognized Babe for the tremendous athlete she was, not the prim and proper woman she wasn't. "She is an incredible human being," he wrote. "She is beyond all belief until you see her perform. Then you finally understand that you are looking at the most flawless section of muscle harmony, of complete mental and physical coordination the world of sport has ever known. There is only one Babe Didrikson, and there has never been another in her class—even close to her class."

ROBIN ARZÓN
ULTRAMARATHONER

"For me, strength is that inner knowing that I can always choose to get up again."

CHAPTER 7

BREAKING INTO THE BOYS' CLUB:
RUNNING TOWARD OPPORTUNITY

By the 1960s, the cult of domesticity was starting to crumble. Being ladylike was still a thing, but the definition was broadening. The birth-control pill offered unprecedented access to freedom, and many Americans were sympathetic to feminist ideas: equal pay for equal work, shared responsibilities in a household, and opportunities for women to serve in managerial roles.

When it came to physical ability, twenty years earlier, World War II had proven that women could keep their homes *and* the home front humming, as Rosie the Riveter said, and the All-American Girls Professional Baseball League demonstrated that women could be entertaining athletes who were powerful, quick, and scrappy. (Even with their satin skirts and oft-reapplied lipstick.) And miracle of miracles, in 1960, the women's 800-meter race returned to the Olympics for the first time since the 1928 race scandalized those who thought women were too delicate to run more than a sprint.

But the march of progress happens only so fast. The majority of people believed there were things men could do that women just couldn't—or shouldn't. While running the 800 meters was accepted by this time, the world wasn't entirely ready for anything significantly longer.

• • •

EVEN IF YOU DON'T RECOGNIZE the name Kathrine Switzer, you've probably seen an image of her. There's an iconic series of shots from the Boston Marathon in 1967 that show race official Jock Semple lunging at her, trying to pull the bib from her sweatshirt and push her off the course. "Give me those numbers and get the hell out of my race!" he screamed.

Switzer was the first female to run the Boston Marathon as an official entrant, but she wasn't trying to circumvent the rules. Nothing on the entry form said it was for men only, and when she signed up, she wrote her name as K. V. Switzer, the same way she'd been writing her name since she was twelve. (She wanted to be a sportswriter, and using initials in the vein of cool writers such as T. S. Eliot and J. D. Salinger seemed like the way to go. It also stopped people from asking her why Kathrine was missing an "e.")

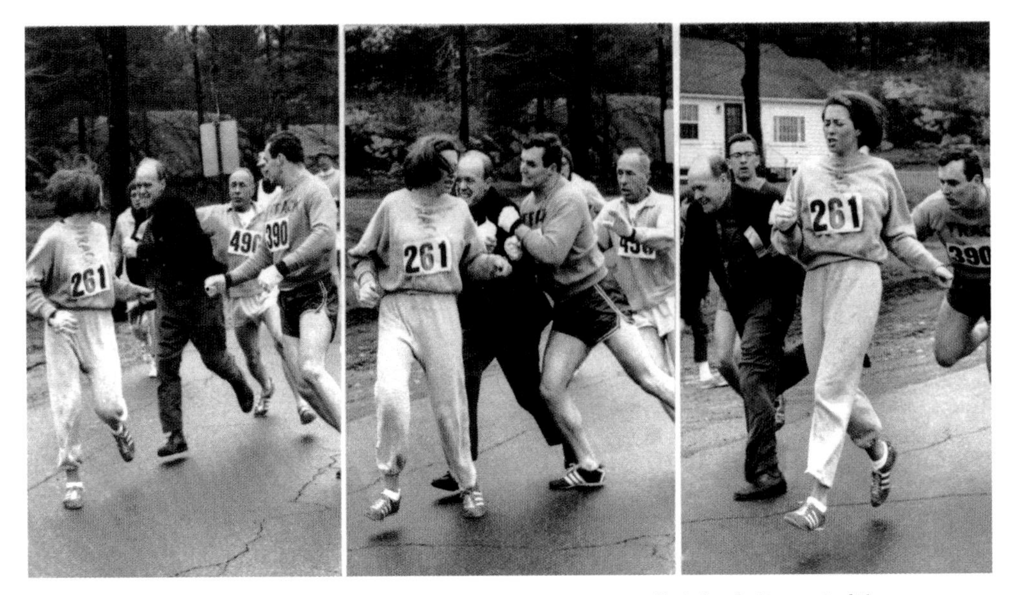

At the 1967 Boston Marathon, official Jock Semple attempts to get Kathrine Switzer out of the race.

A woman named Bobbi Gibb had run the marathon before but only in an unofficial capacity. In 1966, she had taken cover in a forsythia bush near the start line and disguised herself in a hoodie and men's shorts. There was plenty of skepticism about whether she was actually covering the full distance, as many people simply didn't think it was possible for a woman to run 26.2 miles. Even if it was possible, it certainly wasn't safe.

"Women were deemed fragile, incapable of doing difficult things," Switzer says. "The marathon smacked them as the ultimate hard thing. To look exhausted or sweaty in public wasn't a thing a woman would do." Even Switzer's male running partner, who'd been logging some serious mileage with her on a regular basis, didn't think she (or any woman) had what it took.

She did. Although she briefly considered dropping out after the hubbub happened with Semple (who was bodychecked by Switzer's 235-pound boyfriend before he could pull her off the course) just four miles into the race, she knew that if she quit, it would just prove the point that so many already believed, that women weren't cut out for this. She turned the fear and humiliation into anger and pressed on, crossing the finish line with her feet covered in squishy, bloodied blisters but her self-respect intact. (A year later, Semple told *Sports Illustrated* he wasn't opposed to women running longer distances, but he believed in following the rules—and keeping the sexes separate. "I'm in favor of makin' their races longer, but they doon't belong with men," the Scotsman said. "They doon't belong runnin' with Jim Ryun. You wouldn't like to see a woman runnin' with Jim Ryun, wouldya?")

SWITZER'S RUNNIN' CAREER ALL STARTED when, as a twelve-year-old, she told her family she wanted to become a cheerleader. While cheer teams today are often made up of strong, agile athletes capable of performing gymnastics-inspired stunts, such was not usually the case back then. Her dad had other ideas. "You don't want to be a cheerleader," he said. "You shouldn't be on the sidelines cheering for other people. People should cheer for you.... The real game is on the field. Life is for participating, not spectating." He suggested field hockey instead and encouraged his daughter to run a mile around the yard every day to get ready for tryouts.

It sounded crazy, but she took his advice. That summer, the milkman and the mailman saw her running in circles and knocked on the door to ask her mother if she was OK. A girl jogging for the fun of it wasn't standard in the 1950s. Her friends warned her that she might get big legs or a mustache—that's what their parents told them—but instead of facial hair, she gained a "secret weapon." Running not only got her in great shape for playing field hockey, but it transformed her life. "The mile a day was like magic because it changed everything," she says. "It was like a secret armor that was my victory under my belt every day that no one could take away from me. If I got in a difficult situation, I could always say to myself, 'You ran a mile today and he didn't.' "

NOT EVERYONE WAS ENTRANCED BY the magic of Switzer's running. Shortly after the Boston Marathon, race director Will Cloney told reporters, "I am hurt to think that an American girl would go where she is not wanted" and "If that girl were my daughter, I would spank her." As a result of signing up for the Boston Marathon, twenty-year-old Switzer was kicked out of the Amateur Athletic Union (AAU, then the governing body of the sport) for the following reasons:

1. Running a distance of more than one and a half miles, the "longest distance allowable for women."

2. Fraudulently entering the race by signing the entry form with initials.

3. Running the Boston Marathon with men.

4. Running the Boston Marathon without a chaperone.

The adversity fueled her. Switzer went on to finish many more marathons (and was later reinstated by the AAU), eventually running the Boston Marathon in a time of 2 hours, 51 minutes (that's a 6:31-mile pace) and winning the New York City Marathon on a sweltering day by 27 minutes, the biggest margin of victory ever.

Now in her seventies, Switzer believes women will soon outpace men in endurance events. In fact, they already do in some cases. In January 2019, British ultrarunner Jasmin Paris won the coed 268-mile Montane Spine Race, smashing the course record by twelve hours. Following an unforgiving route through Pennine Way, known as the backbone of England, this ultramarathon is considered Britain's most brutal. It features winter weather (think 50-mph winds, rain, and darkness two-thirds of the time), sleep deprivation that would make Madame Anderson proud (Paris logged about three hours total), and nearly 40,000 feet of climbing. Participants must carry the gear they need, including a sleeping bag, a cooking stove, a GPS, a tent/bivouac, and at least 3,000 calories between each of the five checkpoints.

Paris won the race handily; the closest finisher was 15 hours behind her record-breaking time of 83 hours, 12 minutes, and 23 seconds. The small-animal veterinarian, who was working on completing her doctorate at the time of her win, doesn't even consider herself a professional athlete. "I think of it as a hobby," she says. "It's a way of releasing stress. I love to be out in the hills and the mountains—it's just a way of getting out there and feeling free."

All this would make her victory noteworthy enough, but there's more to the story: during the race, she was pumping breast milk at the aid stations.

Avoiding mastitis was the goal for Paris, mother of a then-fourteen-month-old daughter. While it slowed her down a bit, she used those juggling skills parents know so well to make it a nonfactor. "In something like this, any extra thing that you have to do can be a disadvantage, but I managed to be quite efficient," she says. "It's just one of the things on my list I had to do: get food, pick up new maps, express milk."

It isn't only in endurance sports where women shine. On the golf course, men consistently hit the ball faster and farther, but women are more accurate, landing on the fairway a higher percentage of the time. Is a big drive better than finesse, or are they just two equally impressive skills?

"We're really on the cusp of another revolution of breakthrough for women showing that, you know, women do not have the speed and the strength and the power of men, we know that, but what we do have is more endurance, stamina, flexibility, and balance," Switzer says. "For three thousand years of Olympic sport, it's always been about speed, power, strength, but now we're seeing what women can do. As the women have been allowed to emerge, because they've had opportunities to have birth control, and we have modern devices to wash clothes and refrigerators to keep our food—we don't have to be slaves to the domestic burdens of childhood and home—we can be athletes. We're now discovering what women's capabilities are naturally."

The measuring stick for athletic ability is so often tied to power and speed, both traits that are significantly enhanced by muscle mass. And what kinds of sports value power and speed? Nearly all the ones we recognize as most popular: football, basketball, baseball, ice hockey, sprinting, short-distance swimming, rugby . . . the list goes on. These sports have been developed for men and adopted by women, many of whom perform admirably and competitively at them. But what if we changed the paradigm of sports entirely? What if our idea that men are better athletes simply lies in the fact that what we view as athletic is tailor-made for men's abilities?

Switzer has spent time talking to New Zealand's top male endurance runners, and they say that for the longer races, it's the women who carry the team home. That's not just because they have the stamina to keep going but because they're able to maintain a clear head. When the men can no longer read a compass, the women retain their cognitive faculties.

"I don't know what that means," Switzer says, "but I think what's very exciting is maybe sports of the future are going to be looking entirely different from the way they have ever looked in the past, because women are going to be stepping up and creating events that you and I can't even imagine right now."

THERE HAD BEEN A TIME when women weren't considered so weak—at least, not to the extent that they were when Switzer flexed her muscles on the marathon course.

Before the Industrial Revolution shifted large swaths of the population to cities, most people in Europe and North America lived in rural communities. They grew their own food, sewed their own clothes, and crafted their own furniture. Men and women were both farm strong.

Then, at a rapid pace, machines were developed to do the jobs people used to do, in a fraction of the time. Suddenly, people could think about leisure. They no longer had to be completely self-sustaining, which left them with some extra time. (This is one of the reasons Madame Anderson's sport of pedestrianism is said to have attracted such crowds. People had the time to spare, and not a lot of competing activities were yet up and running.) They were also growing more sedentary. Without all those laborious chores to take care of, their muscles weakened, and they didn't need a Fitbit to tell them their daily step count had diminished.

This softness that crept into modern life struck many as problematic, and in the mid-1800s, it led to a movement that's still rippling into today: muscular Christianity.

In earlier days of Christianity, a fit body wasn't much of a concern. In fact, Martin Luther of Protestant Reformation fame thought the Greeks' idea of *mens sana in corpore sano* ("a healthy mind in a healthy body") was just a load of paganism.

But as postindustrial life got easier in many respects, cultural observers wondered if men had become too effeminate. "The emerging crop of Victorian gentlemen had the *gentle* part of their moniker down, but hadn't much to speak of as to the *man* part of the equation," write Brett and Kate McKay, who run the website ArtofManliness.com. "In being excessively high-minded, they had lost touch with the practical realities of life; they could button up their collars but not roll up their sleeves."

At the same time, church services were dominated by women, and Christian leaders wondered how to get more men involved. By tying religion and manhood together, they could kill two birds with one stone, producing men who were stronger and more virile, capable of defending themselves and their country if need be, while also drawing them to the church.

This led to the founding of the Young Men's Christian Association (YMCA) in 1844. Initially, the Y served as a place for guys to attend Bible study and get off the mean streets of London, but as time went on, facilities began adding gyms and swimming pools, combining worship services, living quarters, and recreation options into one package.

Although the founding of the Young Women's Christian Association wasn't far behind, its focus was somewhat different from the YMCA's, without the emphasis on exercise. However, some of the locations were progressive. The Boston YWCA installed pulley weights on the backs of closet doors in 1870 and offered a calisthenics class later that decade. Despite that, entertaining the possibility that muscular Christianity really should apply to both sexes was not a popular opinion.

"For muscle and manhood run together by nature," wrote journalist Eliza Archard in the *Herald of Health*. "But who ever heard of muscular womanhood?"

Prominent men such as Theodore Roosevelt, U.S. president from 1901 to 1909, grew up in this tradition of muscular Christianity, in which sports were a virtuous pursuit that intertwined effort and character. That goes a long way in explaining why he once said of his sons, "I would rather one of them should die than have them grow up weaklings."

It's difficult to imagine anyone saying this about their daughters, but boys and girls have long had different expectations. Whether women have been seen in opposition or as complementary to men, either way, their roles have been defined by what men are not. Consider the following (often unspoken) assumptions:

- Men are masculine. Women are feminine.
- Men are leaders. Women are supporters.
- Men are logical. Women are emotional.
- Men are aggressive. Women are passive.
- Men are providers. Women are nurturers.
- Men are competitive. Women are collaborative.

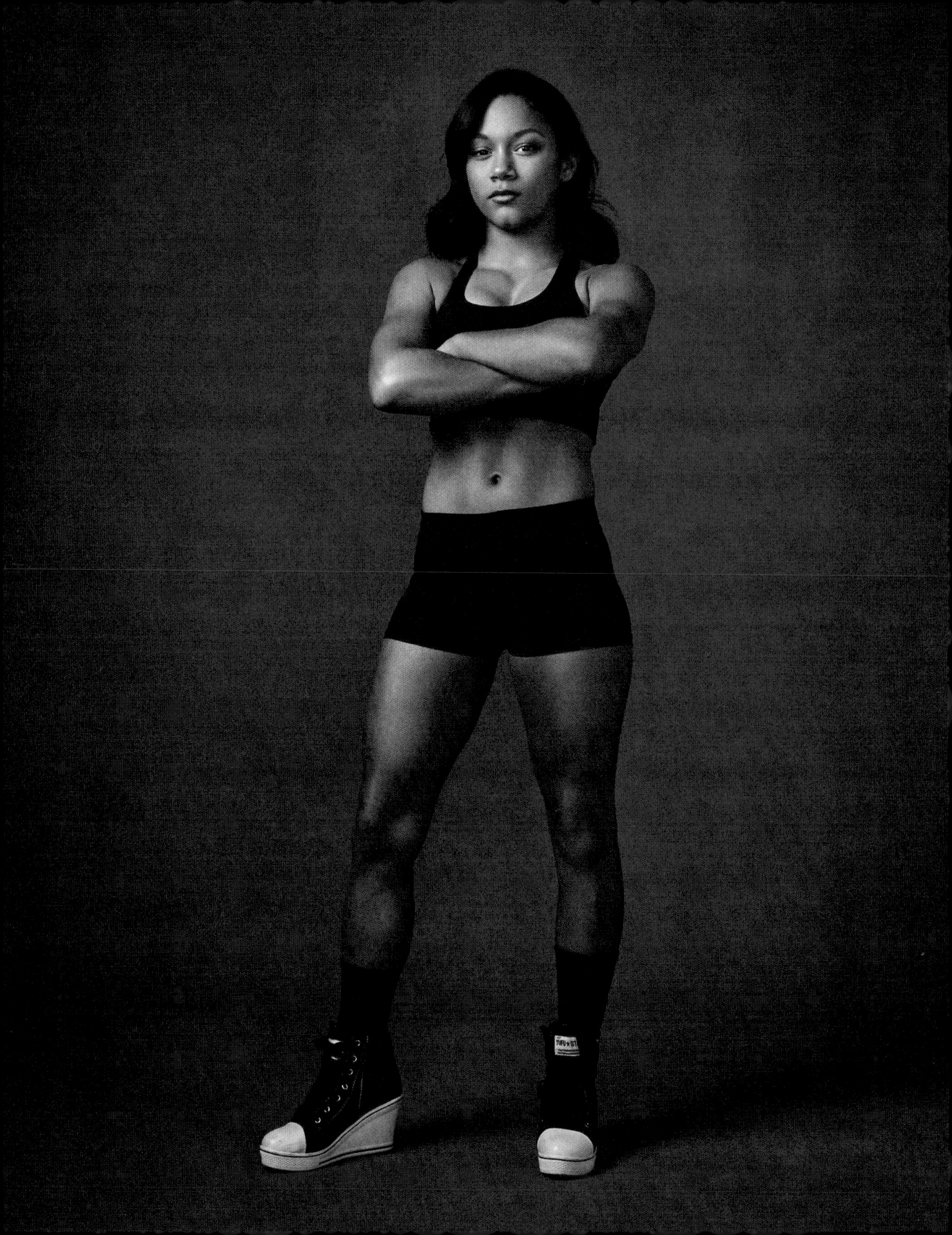

"AFTER I WON THE STATE MEET IN POWERLIFTING AND BEAT ALL THE BOYS, I HAD PEOPLE BOOING ME. THEY DIDN'T LIKE THE FACT THAT I WAS DIFFERENT. IT JUST MADE ME WANT TO WORK HARDER TO SHOW THEM WHO I AM."

DAMIYAH SMITH

ALL-AROUND ATHLETE

- Men are tough. Women are gentle.
- Men are strong. Women are weak.

It's a concept known as gender polarization, and psychologist Sandra Bem said that when we look through a lens in which men and women are mutually exclusive, it permeates all areas of our lives, from what we wear to how we express emotion.

Teddy Roosevelt might not have believed this, but overall, girls and boys share about 99.8 percent of their genes. "There are basic behavioral differences between the sexes, but we should note that these differences increase with age because our children's intellectual biases are being exaggerated and intensified by our gendered culture," neuroscientist Lise Eliot, author of *Pink Brain, Blue Brain,* told the *Observer.* "Children don't inherit intellectual differences. They learn them. They are a result of what we expect a boy or a girl to be."

ONE OF THE PROBLEMS WITH viewing men and women as polar opposites is that men have long been considered the standard, while women are "other," and the standard can, at times, feel like the superior. This plays out in a lot of ways. In referring to body composition, we say women have extra fat but not that men have extra muscle. We do most of our scientific studies on men and then extrapolate the results to women. For example, most crash-test dummies are modeled on the anatomy of the average male, so the safety features are designed with those proportions in mind—as a result, women are 47 percent more likely to be seriously injured in a car accident, even when factors such as height, weight, seatbelt usage, and crash intensity are controlled for. A man is a Mr. his entire life; a woman is a Miss or a Mrs. or a Ms., depending on her marital status—or refusal to define herself in such a way.

Our words almost always default to the masculine form, with a prefix or suffix added for the feminine alternative. *Actor* is standard; *actress* is other. We might call something "man-made" and mean that it's made by a person (a hu*man*, if you will)—because *man* is standard and *woman* is other. If you see a news story about the Final Four, that's assumed to be the men's game; the women's tournament is always marked as such. At my high school, my sports teams were called the Lady Trojans, while the boys' teams were simply the Trojans, not the Gentleman Trojans.

That sets up a dichotomy between men and women that needn't exist. In Teddy Roosevelt's time, the prevailing attitude was that men and women occupied separate spheres. The divide between the sexes became as wide as the corset was narrow.

A century later, that idea nearly kept Switzer and her contemporaries out of the world's most prestigious marathon and added pressure for those who dared to expand a woman's role. There was an unspoken agreement among the early female runners that they would look good while competing and, above all, finish every race they started. Any little misstep could set their cause back, a scary thing to contemplate in a sport where it's all too easy to get dehydrated or twist an ankle. They knew they had to show that they were capable within a framework of femininity, or they might never get another chance to prove how strong they really were.

EVEN TODAY, IN A TIME when gender-neutral names are on the rise and there's more awareness around babies who are intersex (roughly 1 in 1,666 births don't fit neatly into the XX or XY categories), we're still pretty preoccupied with sex—

note the ubiquity of gender-reveal parties, which barely existed ten years ago. They rely heavily on the blue-versus-pink color scheme and come with themes like "Tutus or Touchdowns" and "Cheer Bows or Free Throws."

Many parents have found that their boys have always liked trucks and their girls have always liked dolls, even when they didn't push gendered toys on them. Be that as it may, there are very subtle ways we treat boys and girls differently, and putting them into categories like "wheels versus heels" while releasing a cavalcade of gender-conforming confetti before they're even born plays into that.

"Kids rise or fall according to what we believe about them," neuroscientist Eliot writes, "and the more we dwell on the differences between boys and girls, the likelier such stereotypes are to crystallize into children's self-perceptions and self-fulfilling prophecies."

Most parents think kids should try activities that are typically associated with the opposite sex, according to a recent study from the Pew Research Center, but the percentages did vary significantly based on whether it was girls or boys being discussed. A majority of women (80 percent) and men (72 percent) said it was a good thing for parents of young girls to expose them to so-called boy activities; 9 percent fewer women and 16 percent fewer men said parents of young boys should encourage exploration of girl-oriented activities.

BY TAKING UP JOGGING, MORE traditionally a boys' activity, Switzer received plenty of words of caution. "Girls who ventured out into sports were immediately warned about things," she says. "When I was young, the ones I heard most were you're going to get big legs, you'll never be able to have children—specifically your uterus would collapse or fall out—and you would take on other masculine qualities like grow a beard or get hair on your chest."

She pressed on anyway, and other women joined her in defying gender stereotypes. The most famous example in this era was the "Battle of the Sexes" tennis match in 1973 between Billie Jean King and her bet-loving, lady-bashing foe, retired pro tennis player Bobby Riggs.

Riggs argued that women didn't deserve the same prize money as men, because they were only "about 25 percent as good as men." And really, they shouldn't be on the tennis court at all. To prove his point, he offered $100,000 to any woman who could beat him, assuming that one never would. "Women belong in the bedroom and the kitchen, in that order," he said (many times, in many ways). Some laughed at him, but many laughed with him.

Sportswriters largely came out in support of Riggs, who was a 5-2 favorite to beat King. In the '70s, as the situation still is now, most sportswriters were men. *USA Today* founding editor Nancy Woodhull called them out. "In all their jock mentality, the sportswriters have rallied around Riggs, putting him on a pedestal," she wrote. "Not because he has shown any masculine courage, but because he serves as a reminder of the day when men ruled the world and women kept it clean."

Riggs maintained that King would "crack up" during the match since she was subject to the emotional frailties of the weaker sex. He was wrong, of course. King beat him in straight sets, humbling the antifeminist hustler. Riggs even softened a bit—a very small bit—when he admitted, "I said a lot of things about which I was wrong. Now I have to sit back and take what's coming, and I will. I still like women in the bedrooms and kitchens, in that order, but some of them can do other things."

NO ONE LIKES TO LOSE, BUT THERE'S a difference between wanting to be the victor and being so tied to the idea that men are physically superior to women that it causes a crisis of masculinity if that deeply held belief is challenged.

When Ann Trason competed in a twenty-four-hour mixed-gender ultrarunning championship in 1989, some men said they'd rather die than let her pass them, and eventually, that happened (the passing, not the dying), as Trason won.

Fast-forward to today, and there's still some of that "boys rule, girls drool" attitude floating around in grown-up form, according to former gymnast and current *American Ninja Warrior* competitor Barclay Stockett. "I still hear people be like, 'Oh, you gonna let that girl beat you?' It's this thing that causes men to just puff up their chest, like, 'I'm so much better than a girl.' It's unfortunate that kind of language is still used today, and even amongst adults—we're the examples for children."

Before Stockett was even born, Sylvia Pressler, a hearing officer who ruled in 1973 that Little League needed to open its doors to all children, recognized the benefits for both sexes. "The sooner little boys begin to realize that there are many areas of life in which girls are their equal and that it is no great shame, no great burden to be bested by a girl," she said, "then perhaps . . . we come that much closer to the legislative ideal of sexual equality as well as to relieving a source of emotional difficulty for men."

If we choose not to view men and women in such a binary way, if we don't buy into gender polarization, if we don't support the dichotomy of "free throws or cheer bows," then we allow all people to cultivate strength. Switzer is both an amazing runner and a woman—there is no division there, no double life. Acknowledging this fact doesn't mean there aren't differences between the sexes and that we can't recognize those differences, but strength is no more masculine than vulnerability is feminine. As University of Iowa sports sociologist Susan

Birrell astutely noted, “It’s a short leap from seeing men as physically superior to seeing men as superior, period.”

If Teddy Roosevelt were here now, I’d tell him that we should hope that both our sons and daughters grow up to be strong, not because we fear they’ll be viewed as weaklings but because with physical strength comes that “secret weapon” Switzer spoke of, empowerment, and that’s a gender-neutral concept.

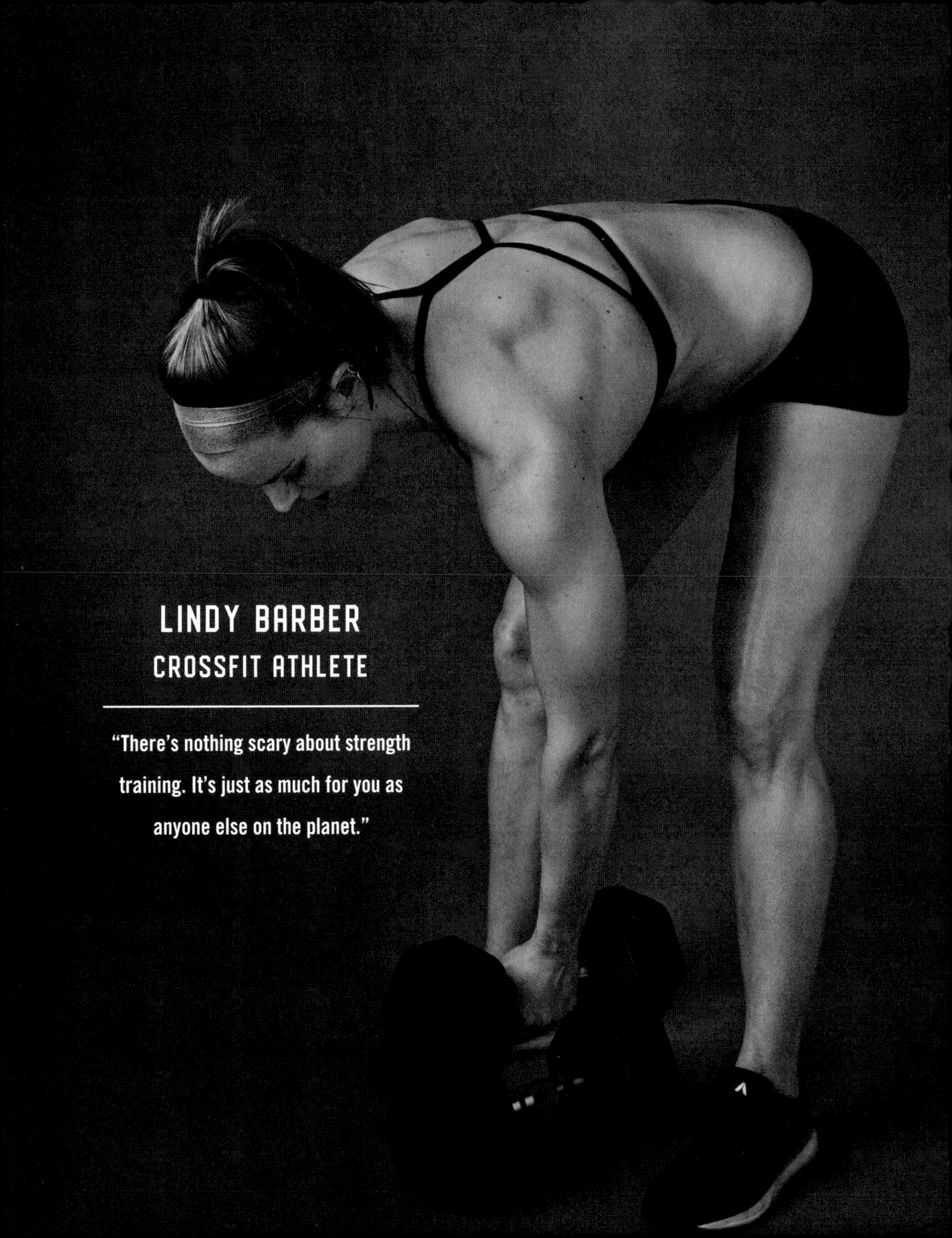

LINDY BARBER
CROSSFIT ATHLETE

"There's nothing scary about strength training. It's just as much for you as anyone else on the planet."

CHAPTER 8

A WOMAN'S PLACE IS IN THE WEIGHT ROOM:

THE RISE OF STRENGTH SPORTS IN THE '70S

During a sports match, there's often a turning point when the momentum shifts. In basketball, it might be a stolen ball that leads to a fast break and ignites one team to come from behind, or in softball, a home run with the bases loaded that makes the players feel unstoppable. In the Calydonian Boar hunt from Greek mythology, it was Atalanta piercing the giant creature behind its ear with an arrow, just as it was about to escape into the woods. That gave fellow hunter Meleager the opening to finish the job with a javelin, putting an end to the boar's terrifying reign and cementing Atalanta's legacy.

The 1970s was one of those turning points. The barriers between men and women that had been crystallized by the muscular Christianity movement were breaking down at record speed. In 1971, girls finally got to play a real, five-player, full-court basketball game. In 1972, women could enter the Boston Marathon without fear of being pushed off the course by an organizer. In 1973, Billie Jean King shut Bobby Riggs up. In 1977, Janet Guthrie was the first woman to race in the Indianapolis 500. Every year, something was happening to advance the notion that girls deserved to get in the game, too.

Arguably, the most notable development came in the form of legislation. When the U.S. Congress passed Title IX of the Education Amendments of 1972, better known simply as Title IX, it prohibited gender discrimination at educational institutions that received federal funds. While this opened doors for women to pursue advanced degrees, it's largely known today for the impact it had on sports at the junior high and high school levels. No longer could public schools devote all their resources to boys' programs. Girls had to be given equal practice facilities, equipment, uniforms, locker rooms, quality of coaching, and publicity, among many other things. In 1972, one in twenty-seven high school girls played a sport. By 1978, that figure had ballooned to one in four.

As doors were flying open left and right, some women decided to press their luck and knock on the still-closed doors of one very intimidating place: the weight room.

LIKE AN EXCLUSIVE MEMBERS-ONLY CLUB, weight rooms in the '70s almost required the invitation of someone who was already on the inside. For the few women who did dare to step among the barbells and squat racks, it was usually a man's introduction that got them in. That was the case for Jan Suffolk, who was an undergrad student at Mercer University excelling in a spontaneous game of log tossing (because don't we all toss logs for fun?) when she caught the eye of a young associate professor.

It was a fitting way to meet for two very strong people. During her senior year in 1973, Jan would marry that professor, Terry Todd, who just happened to be the winner of the super heavyweight division in the first-ever national powerlifting championships nine years earlier.

Jan had always been athletic, but it wasn't until after the wedding that she started tagging along to Terry's workouts. She was bored by the light routines she first tried, but under his tutelage, she started to lift heavy—and realized she was capable of so much more than she had ever imagined.

STRENGTH CHALLENGES SEEM TO HOLD a place in every culture. For centuries in Scotland, it was a heavy granite stone that stood in the space between a boy and a man. Known as *clach cuid fir*, Gaelic for "manhood stone," these boulders usually came from the river, where they'd been buffed and shaped over time by the swirling waters. When a boy was ready to prove that he was fit to enter the ranks of adulthood, he'd take his village's stone—it might be at the castle or the town square—and, in front of his chieftain, lift it from the ground to the top of a wall. Once successful, he was declared a man and got to wear an eagle's feather in his cap.

In 1979, Jan Todd was not a boy on a quest to become a man, but that didn't mean she didn't have something to prove. By this point, she'd become a champion in powerlifting, a sport that tests raw strength in three lifts: squat, bench press, and deadlift. During her first competition in 1975—which she had to petition to be allowed to take part in, since there were no contests for women—she broke a Guinness World Record for the two-hand deadlift that had stood strong for forty-nine years, picking up 394.5 pounds. That record was merely the first of many. The next year, she managed to deadlift more than 400 pounds. She also hit that mark in her squat, and by 1981, she could squat 545.5 pounds.

Terry had told Jan about Scotland's tradition of strength stones. It sounded intriguing—and like a great challenge. In reading a book on the Scottish Highland Games, the couple learned of the most famous example of all: the Dinnie Stones. While most manhood stones weighed somewhere in the neighborhood of 200 pounds, the Dinnie Stones were two slabs of granite that weighed a total of 332.49 kilograms, more than 730 pounds. The unusual shape and uneven size required an awkward split stance when lifting, with one leg stretched forward and the other reaching back.

They were named after Donald Dinnie, a Scottish sporting superstar from the latter half of the nineteenth century. He and his father employed the stones to anchor a roped plank they were using to repair the Potarch Bridge. Legend has it that Dinnie could not only lift these stones simultaneously, but he also walked the width of the bridge with them in hand. (Each has an iron rung for handling.)

Hardly any men had successfully lifted the Dinnie Stones, and certainly no women, but Jan didn't let that deter her. She was determined to try.

TO PREPARE HERSELF FOR THE Herculean task ahead (or perhaps "Atalantan" is more fitting), Jan practiced with barbells at home, doing her best to replicate what picking up the boulders would be like. When the big day came and she arrived at the Old Potarch Hotel, where the stones lived, it was clear the feat would be even more difficult than she had imagined.

"The two brutal-looking rocks were chained together, and as I looked at them closely I began to fear . . . that she might fail to lift them," Terry Todd wrote. "They were much larger than photographs had made them seem, and I knew this would force Jan to take a wider stance than would provide ideal, or even reasonably good, leverage."

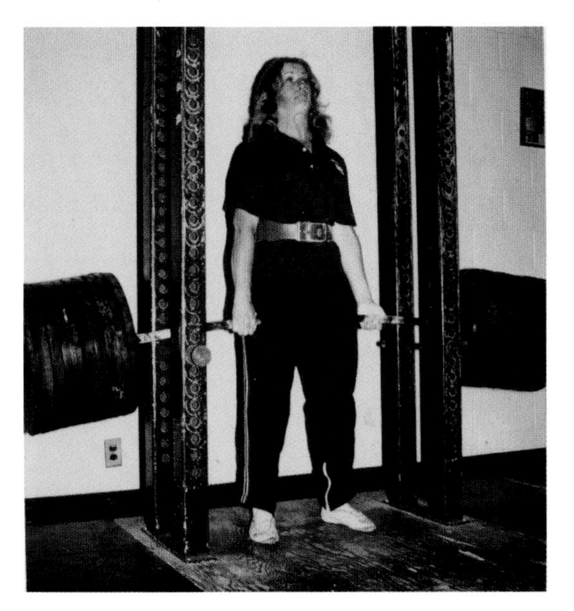

Jan Todd performs an assisted deadlift of more than 1,000 pounds.

The night before the attempt, Jan, Terry, and a couple of friends were taken to the home of a whisky distributor who'd heard about their mission in visiting Scotland. He presented all the men with a bottle of Scotch whisky, conspicuously leaving Jan out. He then presented everyone with a small knife—except, of course, for Jan. "We soon left, realizing as we did so that perhaps everyone in Scotland wasn't as pleased about our primary business there," Terry wrote.

The next morning, Jan prepared for the challenge. Warming up with the stones one at a time was no problem. Jan lifted each one twice with each hand. But when she straddled the stones and tried to pull both at the same time, only the smaller of the two left the ground. A second attempt ended the same way.

She walked down to the River Dee to clear her head. She'd come all this way, she'd trained for months, and she wanted to break this barrier not only for herself but also for other women. If she could do it, so could someone else. This could bust down the macho doors of the weight room, open the floodgates for women who felt limited by what they'd been told they could achieve. Setting this example might just change some perspectives, maybe even lives.

As Jan got ready for a third go, Terry leaned in and whispered, "Let's see you pull this one for the whisky man."

This time, Jan pulled, her face flushed, her body braced, her expression one of steely determination. The smaller stone swung off the ground ("smaller" being a relative term for something 300-plus pounds), and ever so slowly, the larger stone cleared, too. It was only for a moment, but the task was complete. According to the Scottish rite of passage, she was officially a wo(man)—one certainly deserving of a celebratory dram of whisky.

THE GRANDDADDY OF ALL STRENGTH sports is weightlifting, with origins that date back to ancient Greece, China, and Egypt. It appeared on the docket at the first modern Olympic Games in 1896 and has been contested at each Olympics since 1920. (On the men's side, that is. Women didn't get the chance to throw down on the Olympic stage until the beginning of this century.)

While weightlifting does involve lifting weights, it's a little more technical than that. The sport centers around the Olympic lifts, known as the "clean and

“WHEN YOU FEEL LIKE THROWING IN THE TOWEL, ASK YOURSELF, ‘AM I WHERE I WANT TO BE YET?’ IF THE ANSWER IS NO, KEEP PUSHING FORWARD.”

CAMILLE BROWN

WEIGHTLIFTER

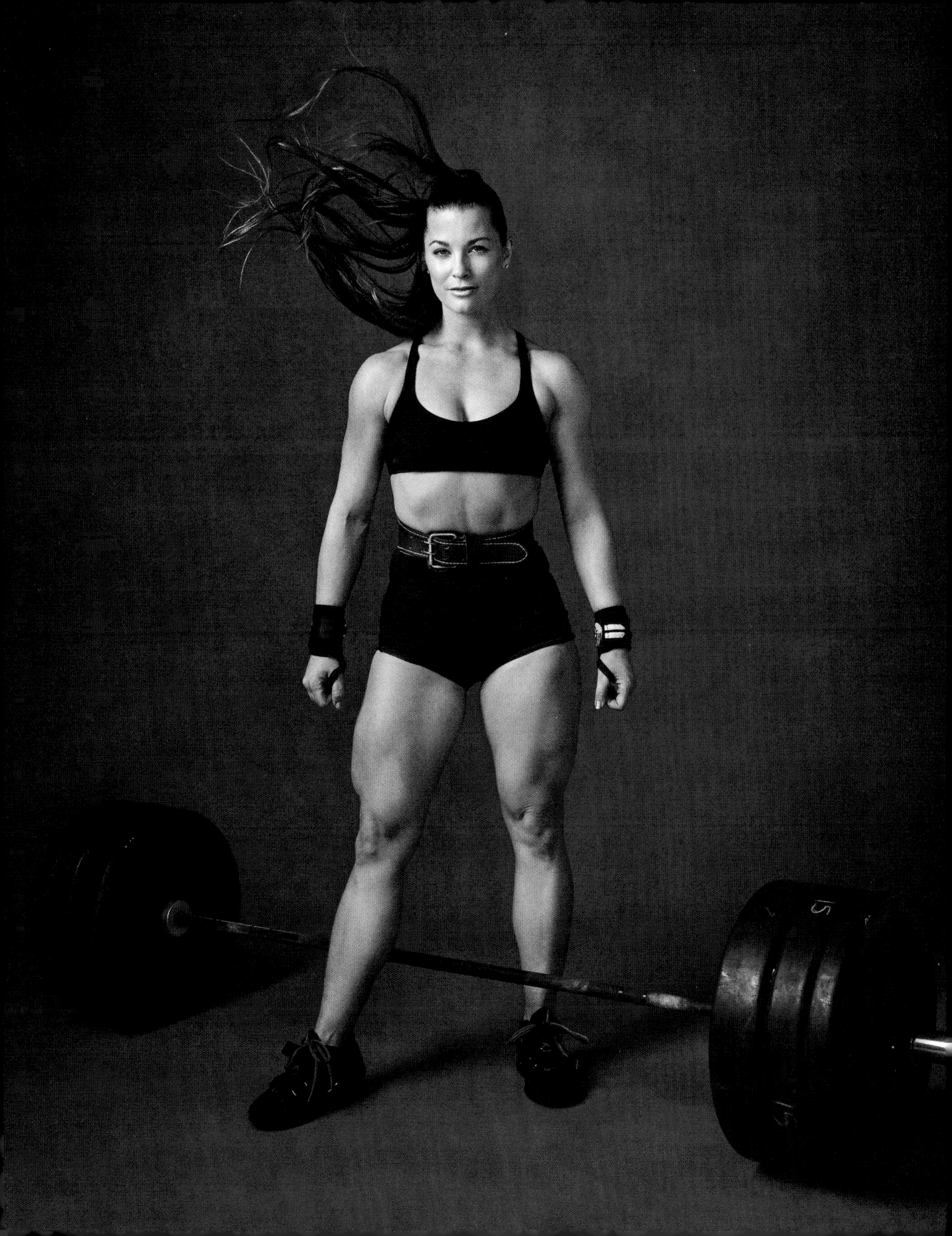

jerk" and the "snatch," which test explosive strength, mobility, speed, and coordination. "To get the weight from the floor to locked arms overhead takes seconds—it's very dynamic," says weightlifter Karyn Marshall.

It was 1978 when Marshall, then a college student, lifted her first barbell in a dark, windowless YMCA basement. (Her introduction was through her boyfriend and his coach.) She found she had a knack for it, and in no time at all, she was posting lifts that rivaled those of some of the men around her. "I just fell in love with it," she says. "I kind of enjoyed the fact that it was a brand-new sport for women and that it involved being strong and being different."

Women's divisions didn't exist, so when she went to enter the all-male regional qualifier for New York's Empire State Games in the spring of 1979, she was initially denied by organizers. Eventually, because it was a small, local meet, they allowed her to compete anyway. She placed first in her weight class and should have successfully qualified for the statewide competition, but because the Empire State Games considered weightlifting a men's-only sport, she was ultimately barred from taking her rightful spot.

She started to wonder whether training to compete was futile. Without a local, national, or international contest for women, how much could she really achieve? She asked her coach if he thought she had the strength to hang with the men. With no hesitation, he responded yes. That boosted her confidence and saw her through to 1981, when women in the U.S. won the right to have a competition of their own—by one vote. The governing body for weightlifting was split 50–50 on whether to go forward with a women's national championship, but the president of the organization broke the tie in favor. Marshall won nine women's national championships, en route to setting forty-five national records, breaking Sandwina's seventy-five-year-old mark for most weight lifted overhead, and becoming the first woman in history to clean and jerk more than 300 pounds.

Six years after competing in a women's event for the first time, Marshall found herself at the inaugural Women's World Weightlifting Championships in Daytona Beach, Florida. The Chinese lifters were surprisingly dominant. Disappointment hung in the air, as in one weight class after another, the U.S. lifters were settling for silvers or bronzes, not what they had expected. On the morning of the final day, the executive director for USA Weightlifting approached Marshall and told her she was the United States' last hope for a gold medal. "I just felt this destiny of 'I'm going to win, don't worry about it,'" she says. "There was this confidence of knowing that's what I had to do."

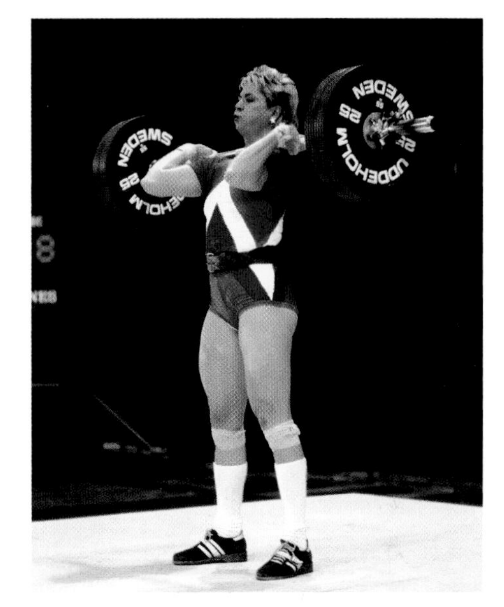

Karyn Marshall sets for a jerk of 120 kilograms (264.5 pounds) at the 1988 U.S. Women's National Weightlifting Championships. She won the 82.5-kilogram class.

She took that attitude to the platform and readied herself. The crowd was silent. She went into a zone of total focus, a head space she'd cultivated through years of relentless training. She bent down to pick up the bar, contracted every muscle in her body, and pulled until the barbell was resting on her shoulders. Next, a knee dip, right leg forward, left leg backward, arms outstretched.

Just like that, 275 pounds was above her head, a smile was on her face, and the gold medal would soon be around her neck.

Now a chiropractor, Marshall says her experiences as a weightlifter carried over into other areas of her life. After she decided to get a doctor of chiropractic degree, she graduated as the valedictorian of her class. "I'm not afraid of hard work," she says. "I'm not afraid to dedicate myself to something very single-mindedly and to put 100 percent effort into it."

That skill set was also helpful when she found herself battling stage 2 breast cancer in 2011. It wasn't just the measurable strength that the former World's Strongest Woman possessed; it was that toughness she developed back when women weren't supposed to lift heavy weights. "Weightlifting's not just about your physical strength. It's a mental game—to push through something that's really hard, then to have the mindset that just because it's hard doesn't mean you can't do it, and not to be afraid of it," she says. "I just tried my best to have a mentality to take it as a challenge and I'm going to do everything I can, and as hard as this is—chemotherapy's really hard—that it was a temporary thing and I'm going to get to the other side and I'm going to be stronger for it."

MUSCLE BEACH'S PUDGY STOCKTON HAD set the example with a barbell. In fact, when Jan Todd started lifting, she looked at pictures of Pudgy for reassurance that she was moving in the right direction. Now these female lifters in the 1970s took her lessons and ran with them, pushing the boundaries of what was possible in a way that would have made supernaturally strong Sandwina proud.

Not only did they have barbells to contend with—which provide an interminable challenge, given that you just increase the weight the stronger you get—but they also had detractors who didn't believe they were worthy of whisky or a spot in a competition. Jan Todd recalled in an interview women who told her humiliating stories of having to weigh in nude in front of the male judges or wear a jockstrap because the rules, which were clearly written for men, mandated it.

There was a big mental hurdle to cross, too. Training in any strength sport requires taking up space, whether it's in a weight room or on a lifting platform. And taking up space can be difficult for women. Just look at any crowded area where men and women are both sitting, and you'll see the women with legs pulled tightly together, while the men are more likely to have their knees wide apart, a phenomenon known as "manspreading." There's debate about whether there are good biological reasons for this behavior, but regardless of whether the width of the pelvis and the angle of the femoral neck really make it harder for a man to keep his legs in line with the width of the seat he's in, I feel confident saying that men worry far less than women do about how much space they're taking up and how others around them might feel about it.

In the 1970s, for some women, the pros of getting strong outweighed the cons of the discomfort of stepping outside the little box they'd been told they should occupy. Their sports remained on the fringes, their passions possibly never understood by their loved ones, and yet they got swole anyway. Jan Todd and Karyn Marshall were not strong for girls, they were just plain strong. Only a minuscule percentage of the male population today could lift the Dinnie Stones or clean and jerk Marshall's best. These women changed the idea of what was possible, inspiring others and ushering in an era where health and fitness were about to enter the collective consciousness in a big way. Soon a male introduction to the weight room wouldn't be de rigueur. The momentum had officially shifted, and now it was a ball rolling down a hill in a way that couldn't be stopped.

"Strength should be an attribute of all humanity," Jan said in 1979. "It's not a gift that belongs solely to the male of the species."

Before Jan picked up the Dinnie Stones, would anyone have ever thought that was within the realm of natural ability for a woman?

Yet, when that final stone swung off the ground, seemingly in slow motion, it encapsulated all the work that had been done that decade—and the decades leading up to it—to show that women were capable of greatness. Society's preconceived notions about what a woman could physically achieve might have seemed ground into place, but, like the Dinnie Stones, with enough effort, they could be lifted.

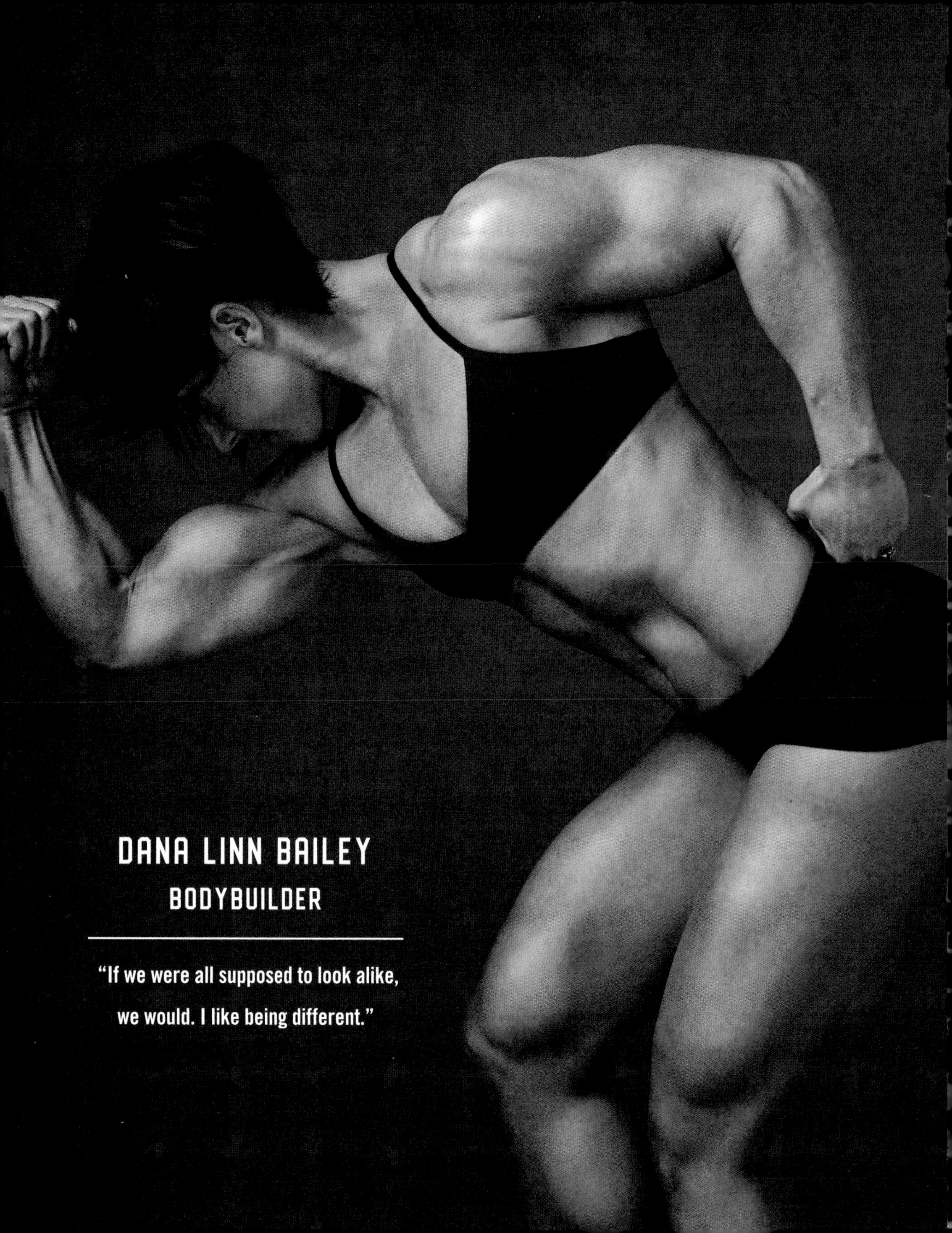

DANA LINN BAILEY

BODYBUILDER

"If we were all supposed to look alike, we would. I like being different."

CHAPTER 9

A BUILT BODY: WHEN MUSCLES ARE REQUIRED TO SHINE

Like powerlifter Jan Todd and weightlifter Karyn Marshall, Elaine Craig found her way inside a weight room in the 1970s with the help of her significant other. As a high school student in California, her football-player boyfriend was always in the gym. If she wanted to see him, she needed to go there, too. She was a track runner and a flag twirler, but lifting weights was not something she ever considered—it was pretty taboo for girls. She was skeptical of the weight room, but her boyfriend put together a routine for her. She decided to give it a shot. If she didn't like it, she wouldn't do it again.

"I had spent all those years running and didn't really see any change in my body, but when I got on that Universal [weight machine], I started seeing this difference happen really fast," she remembers. "I realized how much weightlifting really made a difference."

After graduating from college, she moved to Washington and vividly remembers watching the weather change as she drove up the coast. By the time she reached the Evergreen State, it was raining, and she decided that all the precipitation falling from the sky was not conducive to running. It was time to find a new workout of choice. She joined a health club, met some fitness-minded people, and was introduced to a gym manager who said that if she showed up every day for a week, he'd train her for a bodybuilding show. Back then, the gyms got the glory for successful athletes, and he was looking for a competitor who could win. She thought the woman he'd previously trained was beautiful, so she gave it a go. Her first show was in 1980, and she competed through 1986. She loved it so much that she continues to host bodybuilding competitions with her husband, Brad.

In the early years of their marriage, they owned a gym. When she was out promoting it at fairs at the mall, she'd wear the fitness uniform of the day: a shiny leotard and tights, à la Jane Fonda, which made her look like all the other women who were into aerobics, even though she had some of the biggest biceps in the world at the time at 16.5 inches. "When people would see my pictures, they'd say, 'Oh, gross, who would want to look like that?' And I would say, 'Oh, that's me,' and they'd go, 'That isn't you,' and then I'd flex my biceps," she says. "That was our selling point—well, you can come in and you can do whatever you want and be whatever shape you want."

CRAIG AND OTHER BODYBUILDERS FLEW in the face of what society expected women to look like. Sculpting their bodies into a shape that had traditionally been associated with masculinity was a subversive thing to do. Their actions were saying, "The mainstream standards of beauty don't control my body. I control my body."

In a world in which those who care about female equality usually believe in casting away expectations related to looks, the appearance-based activity of bodybuilding can seem like a contradiction. But when women defy the stereotypes surrounding their bodies and feminine appeal, it can create a space for empowerment.

Bodybuilding is usually considered to have started around 1900 with German-born Eugen Sandow—yes, our old pal who wasn't quite as strong as

Sandwina that one fateful night, as legend has it. A childhood trip to Italy, where he saw sculptures of the athletes of ancient times, convinced him that strength with an eye toward aesthetics was a worthy goal.

Contrary to the prevailing ideas at the time, Sandow didn't believe building a great body was a mission only suitable for men. He was all for women working out. In fact, he found it strange that others didn't recognize the benefits. He encouraged ladies to trade in their corsets and small shoes, which he dubbed "incalculable evils," for comfortable clothes that would improve their health and vigor.

Three-quarters of a century later, the corsets and small shoes were mostly in museums, but not everyone was as enthusiastic about women's bodybuilding as Sandow was.

IN 1977, THE DOCUDRAMA *PUMPING IRON* was released, set in the golden age of men's bodybuilding, when titans like Arnold Schwarzenegger and Lou Ferrigno wowed with their chiseled physiques. The movie was popular, vaulting the niche sport into the public eye, and when women started participating in bigger numbers after the first contest in 1977, filmmakers decided to make a follow-up. *Pumping Iron II* followed the women training for the 1983 Caesars World Cup, who were well aware of the public's skepticism of bodybuilding as a coed sport. Legendary film critic Gene Siskel started his review of the movie this way: "You might expect a documentary about a women's weightlifting competition to be not much more than a freak show."

In a scene filmed in the shower, with some gratuitous shots of soapy side boob, a few bodybuilders chat about the issues they face, such as intimidated men. "I think one of the things that grosses people out about bodybuilders when they flex is these people are seeing muscles on us that they don't even know they have themselves," one competitor says. "And it should be something beautiful to see; it's not gross to see your abs."

The sight of abs can be alarming if you don't know they're in there somewhere (I'm still searching for mine), but to call them gross seems unhelpful. Why were a dedication to fitness and a diet void of junk food considered gross?

"When a woman came out in a two-piece and flexed her biceps, as I used to say, 'on purpose,' or flexed her quads, it shocked people," says Steve Wennerstrom, the women's historian for the International Federation of Bodybuilding (IFBB). "It was just something most people hadn't seen or even thought about."

A frequent writer of strength-training articles, Fred Howell was in this camp. "Like many men, I was at first against women's bodybuilding contests," he wrote. "It was silly, I thought, for a girl to strike a double-biceps pose with nine-inch upper arms. And in the back of my mind, I felt it was just unfeminine."

A skeptical Howell attended his first show and penned an article about it. Backstage, men grumbled about wasting their time and giving "those freaks" space on the stage—space they thought they should be occupying instead.

"Why were they working so hard in the gym?" Howell mused. "Did it make them mannish; were they man-haters; victims of a hormone imbalance; angry at being women? Or were they simply women needing and wanting to exercise—to feel good, look good, and compete in a sport after their school days were over?"

As soon as the women took the stage, he became a convert. The attitude and energy they brought was infectious, as was their competitive desire. They were athletes, full stop. And they were vibrant ones at that. (Of course, Howell had to go and taint his new, informed outlook with this line: "Fear not, fellas, breasts are definitely a feature of the . . . women.")

AS THE PUBLIC WAS EXPOSED to more portrayals of muscular definition on women, the initial shock faded into appreciation. The way these women could mold their bodies was impressive. Many participants found their way to the sport in an effort to lose body fat or gain strength in order to keep up with their kids, and they discovered they liked the way they looked and felt after consistent weight training. The level of muscularity wasn't very high by modern standards, but as the sport progressed and the women got bigger—in some cases, with the help of steroids—it became the target of vitriol again.

But if there was disagreement outside the inner circle of bodybuilding about how muscular a woman should really get, there was even more within its ranks.

Those early days were often fraught. Competitions were confusing, for spectators, judges, and entrants alike, because no one knew what they should be looking for. Even Henry McGhee Jr., the organizer of the first women's bodybuilding contest in the U.S., had trouble explaining his vision, but he was clear that he believed women belonged on the stage.

"Men don't monopolize strength. If they did, you wouldn't see fillies winning horse races. Women are incredible. We've just never seen them reach their potential," he told *Sports Illustrated*. "When I was a high school track coach, the girls would leave the team when they started getting muscular, and that was frustrating to me. I decided that I wanted to promote muscle on women as beautiful. I think that using traditional standards of femininity in a bodybuilding contest is like having a spelling bee only for those spelling on a fifth-grade level or less. We don't know the ultimate potential of women, and already they want to limit it."

Women's bodybuilding historian and sports photojournalist Wennerstrom agreed and was in favor of women packing on as much muscle as they liked. "I was wanting women to realize they should challenge their physicality at whatever level they desired," he says. "The 'femininity' aspect made me crazy because a woman's a woman, no matter what her look is."

The Terminator himself, Arnold Schwarzenegger, has always been in support of women's competitions being just like men's. "Judges sometimes look for the sexiest women, but they should forget that," he said. "People say it's OK to have women onstage, but that they shouldn't pose like men. But the point is for them to demonstrate their physical development, to show it off in a dynamic way, and if someone says, 'It turns me off to see a woman hit a muscular shot,' well, who cares?"

On the other side were people like Doris Barrilleaux, an early organizer of women's bodybuilding shows, who advocated a softer look. She later said she wished they'd called the sport "body sculpting" from the start and that she was dismayed when it trended toward "bigger is better." "I don't want people to think it was my idea to make women look like men," she said. "I don't believe in all this muscle stuff that they're into now." (Interestingly, a photo of Barrilleaux posing with both biceps flexed was rejected in 1962 by *Strength and Health* magazine for not being feminine enough. She sent in a second, of her sitting on the beach, and that was published.)

Mr. America for 1973, Jim Morris, took her point several steps further. He volunteered to judge a 1979 show—perhaps as an act of masochism, because afterward, he had this to say: "I think female physique contests should be discontinued. I'm no more in favor of them than I am of male beauty contests. To me, one is as repulsive as the other."

In the early '80s, the IFBB published guidelines to try to clear up just what judges should be looking for. Muscularity, shape, proportion, symmetry, and presentation—all the same criteria the men had—were chosen. "Femininity is a social concept, not a biological reality," the guidelines read, "and it has little to do with the sport of bodybuilding, any more than female high jumpers or tennis players are required to be 'feminine' in order to compete."

The interpretation of factors such as shape and proportion still left plenty to argue about. Viewers get an inside look at this tension in *Pumping Iron II*, when the judges can't agree on just what the standards should be. One judge says putting a limit on muscularity is like telling a female skier that she can only ski so fast, while an official calls big muscles "grotesque" and insists that they need to turn people on, not off.

THE BATTLE OVER HOW MUCH muscle is too much found its nexus when Rachel McLish and Bev Francis stood next to each other onstage at the 1983 Caesars World Cup. At one end of the spectrum was American McLish, strong and sculpted but with plenty of curves, model good looks, and a glittering, illegally padded bikini top. At the other end, Australian Francis was a world-class powerlifter who brought an epic eight-pack to the stage and a boxy shape that struck many as manly and cartoonish. This moment is captured in *Pumping Iron II*. "With her squat chest, arms, and legs, Bev doesn't look anything like the sinewy sex kitten Rachel McLish," Siskel wrote in his review. "Rachel is more the Incredible Tease to Bev Francis' Incredible Hulk."

"I always felt that I was a little bit different," Francis says in the movie. "I always admired strength—anything, whether it was human or animal or the weather. I loved thunderstorms, anything that's big and strong and powerful. And I always wanted to be powerful myself. . . . I never had the confidence in myself to think that I could be better, to think that I could be the strongest woman in the world or anything like that. It was only later years when I came across others that encouraged me. . . . It was a joy to get stronger."

In today's world of bodybuilding, Francis and McLish wouldn't even enter the same category. While they're really fighting for the same thing—the right for women to train their muscles and show them off—the movie pits them against each other, as if they are polar opposites instead of two sides of the same coin.

• • •

WHATEVER THE RESULTING PROPORTIONS, PURPOSELY trying to fashion one's body into a shape that many still associated with masculinity took some guts. The ones who succeeded in winning competitions were, by and large, the ones who retained some of those conventionally accepted qualities that embodied femininity. The male gaze mattered, as it still does. In today's bikini division, "overall look" is one of the judging criteria. That means your suit, hair, skin tone, makeup, and even nails are up for assessment. In other words, femininity is a judging criterion, even if not overtly stated.

Breast implants are common in bodybuilding circles, given that competitors often get down to such low body-fat levels that they lose the volume in their boobs. To maintain traditionally feminine, pleasing proportions, many choose surgical enhancement or at least feel pressured to consider it.

Modern competitor Dana Linn Bailey faced these issues head-on. "I would go to shows and they would mark me down for being too masculine," she remembers. "I would talk to the judges afterward and they would say, 'Get a boob job and stop lifting so heavy.' " She ignored them. Winning a competition might be dependent on the subjective opinions of a panel of judges, but they couldn't measure what getting strong had brought to her life.

"Luckily I liked benching more than I liked boobs," she says. "I also had an incredible husband who said, 'I like you the way you are and you're perfect the way you are; you don't need to go through surgery and put water balloons under your skin to make you pretty.' I'm not against breast augmentations—everyone needs to make a decision based on their own feelings—but deep down I didn't want them. I would be getting them for someone else's approval, and as soon as you do that, you lose yourself."

Bailey kept her well-defined pecs, and it ended up being the best decision for her. Competitively, sticking to her guns eventually paid off when she won the first-ever IFBB pro card in the newly created physique category in 2011.

"All those things that I was so insecure about are now my best features," she says. "One of my most attractive features is being confident with the lack of chest I have, and people appreciate me and see me as a real person because I'm not a Barbie doll."

The acceptance of visible muscularity, though, is still informed by strong opinions on all sides. When Bailey first started lifting heavy weights fifteen years ago, she felt great, but the unsolicited reactions she received weren't always kind. "Even though I was liking my body, nobody else was liking my body," she says. "I would walk into a restaurant wearing a tank top and people's faces would actually be grossed out at me."

That might have discouraged a younger version of Bailey, the one who was self-conscious about her legs and chest as a teen, but her bodybuilding career gave her more than just well-defined pecs and boulder shoulders. It gave her the self-assurance to be unfazed by others' opinions.

"All the comments have helped me develop a very thick skin that I think has boosted my confidence, if anything," she says. "It helps me to realize it doesn't matter why this person isn't OK with me if I'm OK with me."

Bailey walked in the footsteps of those early competitors, who shocked sensibilities not only by lifting heavy weights but also by actually putting the results on display. It was one thing to develop muscularity as a side effect of playing a sport; it was quite another to actively pursue the look.

SO WHY NOT CHOOSE TO compete in a sport with objective numbers instead of subjective criteria that seem to swing back and forth every year? For some, there's magic in realizing you have some agency in the way your body looks, even if it means being judged against shifting standards.

Craig examined her family tree and saw that her genetic line included ancestors who were overweight and suffered from associated health problems. As fun

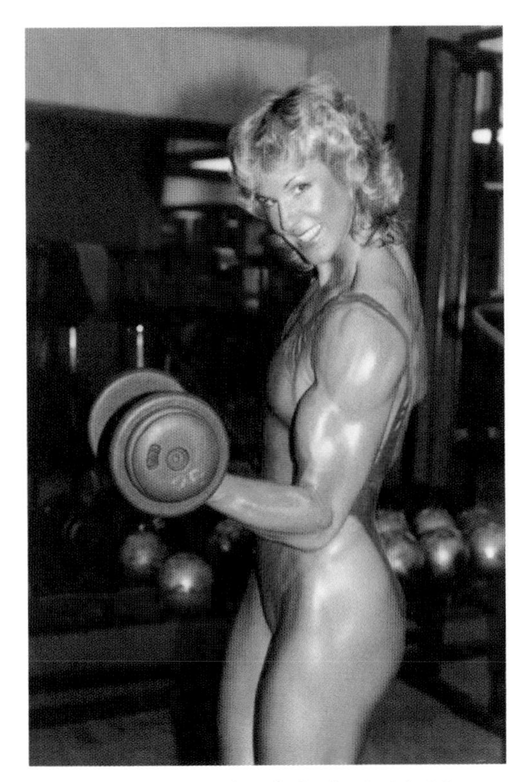
Elaine Craig pumps iron during her bodybuilding career, which began in the early 1980s.

as running and aerobics were, she knew she'd found the antidote to a growing waistline when she discovered lifting. "You do not have to succumb to what your genetics are," she says. "Weight lifting is the magic pill."

Not only does bodybuilding help people reach aesthetic goals, but Craig thinks it's also changed our ideas about aging. Back in 1983, when she was promoting her first show, she brought in a thirty-five-year-old bodybuilder named Georgia Fudge to do some guest posing. As the emcee, twenty-four-year-old Craig kept emphasizing that Fudge was *thirty-five years old.* This seemed practically elderly at the time for a woman to be in incredible shape. Fudge rocked the stage, and the audience went crazy, amazed by what someone so "old" could look like. "That's what weight lifting has done, in my opinion," Craig says. "Good nutrition, health, and getting to the gym has completely changed what thirty-five, forty, forty-five, fifty is."

Despite the progress that's been made from the 1970s until now in terms of accepting a wider set of measurements for women, bodybuilding will likely remain controversial. Any activity where the winner is chosen based on appearance is bound to be contentious, and success is still somewhat tied to presenting an image of femininity. None of that has deterred Craig. She continues to be involved in the sport today because she believes in both the power of lifting weights—it keeps her aches and pains away as she's getting older—and the power of standing under those bright lights. "Once somebody gets onstage, they've accomplished a goal," she says. "They're learning their body and what they can do physically and emotionally and mentally. If you can get up onstage, you can do everything you want to do in life."

JEN WIDERSTROM
FITNESS TRAINER

"What I have to say is greater than anything I've ever looked like."

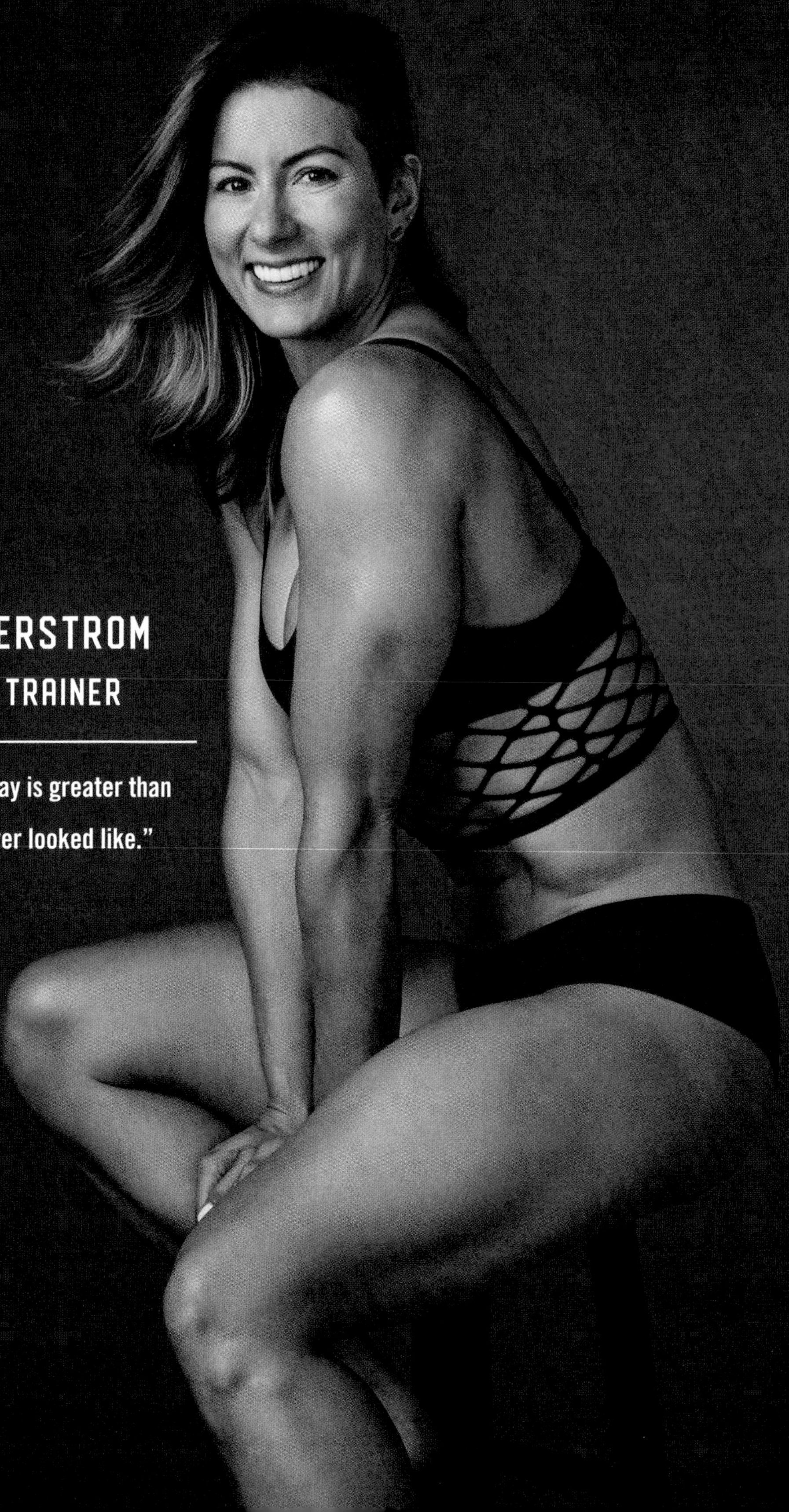

CHAPTER 10

FORM FOLLOWS FUNCTION:
HOW BODY EXPECTATIONS ARE BORN

Bodybuilding is an obvious sport where strength and appearance intersect, but looks have long played a role in the way people feel about strong women. Ada Anderson's rosy cheeks, Sandwina's hourglass figure, Pudgy Stockton's shining skin, Kathrine Switzer's fashionable running outfits, and Elaine Craig's model proportions all made a difference in how they were perceived.

Growing up in Iceland, Katrin Davidsdottir always wanted to be smaller. She was a head taller than all her friends, and in her chosen sport of gymnastics, lithe was the preferred look. "It was a successful day if I could eat less or if I felt light in training. That was a feeling of success for me," she remembers.

After injuring her ankle, she realized that while she enjoyed the discipline and conditioning of gymnastics, she didn't love the sport. She quit and dabbled in track, but it didn't fill that intense training void that gymnastics left, and the competitive fire within her was in search of a place to burn.

Then, when Davidsdottir was eighteen, fellow countrywoman Annie Thorisdottir won the CrossFit Games. It was a big deal for the small island nation, and it opened her eyes to a sport she might want to give a try.

It was love at first WOD (workout of the day, in the vocabulary of CrossFitters). It didn't matter so much anymore that her friends were tiny and she was not built the same way. Now Davidsdottir was in a sport that rewarded all-around athletes, and there were endless new skills to learn and perfect. To be successful, she needed to be able to sprint short distances and run for miles, lift light barbells fast and heavy barbells with power, walk on her hands and jump with her feet, row for two hours and put the pedal to the metal for two minutes. The body that resulted from all those training sessions wasn't created to fit an ideal image; it was forged for utility.

"When I look at how far I've come, and all those hours of diligent work, it makes me so proud," she says. "I'm, like, 'Wow, look at what my body can do, look how fast it can run and how much weight it can lift.' I put my body through so much, and every day it recovers and gets ready for the next day."

Davidsdottir and her very capable body have won the CrossFit Games twice, and she remains in the upper echelon of the sport. Much of her success has come from her mentality and ability to suffer. She likens herself to a sled dog who's happiest when she's putting in serious work.

"I just want everyone to be able to be proud of who they are and what they can do," she says. "We all are so different. I'm not going to be as good at gymnastics as someone else or as strong as someone else, but I at least want to believe that if I put in the work, I can accomplish anything anyone else can do."

She no longer wakes up crossing her fingers that she's lighter than yesterday. While she's an inspiration to many, she's particularly touched by the messages she receives from her youngest fans. When she was growing up, there weren't a lot of muscular role models, and Davidsdottir is proud to be that.

"Little girls come up to me or moms send pictures of them lifting little barbells and doing burpees on the floor," she says. "All they want to do is exercise and be stronger and healthier. I want little girls everywhere to be able to look at me and say, 'If she can accomplish that, I can do that, too.'"

• • •

WHEN DAVIDSDOTTIR APPEARED IN *ESPN* magazine's Body Issue in 2019, an annual special edition that celebrates bodies from a wide range of athletic disciplines, she received a huge outpouring of support, but comments popped up in some corners of the Internet that weren't so complimentary. "She looks like a man from that angle," said one. "Phenomenal athlete, of course, but her build is too developed for me," read another.

Why are muscles on a woman like Davidsdottir something to be criticized and labeled unfeminine? It's a complicated question to answer.

Evolutionary psychology offers some insights into how we determine what someone should look like, although it does a better job of explaining facial beauty than "attractive" bodies. We tend to like faces that are symmetrical, probably because symmetry suggests good genes and youthfulness. (Although we find absolutely perfect symmetry to be creepy, a good reminder that shooting for sheer perfection isn't always the best goal.)

We would recognize a good-looking face as such across eras and cultures, but body types are a different story. If there were a hardwired standard of body-type beauty, it would remain constant, but such a thing doesn't exist. Ancient Egyptians prized narrow shoulders and a high waist, while ancient Greeks favored plump figures with wide hips (and were partial to redheads and blondes). In the past century, the 1920s celebrated flat-chested, petite women, while the 1980s gave us the tall, long-legged supermodel standard. Today it's considered desirable to have toned arms, big breasts, and a full booty.

So what made us think the voluptuous women of Peter Paul Rubens's paintings were beautiful in the 1600s, while tiny Twiggy was all the rage 350 years later—and how does muscle fit in?

For starters, what's difficult is often desirable. Women have been asked to jump through hoops throughout history, so it shouldn't come as a surprise that the more challenging a particular body type is to attain, the more attractive we find it. In periods of famine, plumpness is sought after. In relative times of wealth, thinness rules. In the wake of the Depression, when many didn't have enough to eat, health was associated with having some meat on your bones. The message in an ad run by the Ironized Yeast Company was typical of this time: "Men wouldn't look at me when I was skinny. But since I gained 10 pounds this new, easy way I have all the dates I want."

Bodies are also a way to convey social status. To be fair-skinned in ancient Greece meant you weren't a slave—slaves worked outdoors and developed tans. In Victorian and Edwardian times, that small waist obtained by a tight corset meant you weren't off toiling in a factory or otherwise engaged in manual labor, because it was kind of hard to breathe in them. Instead, you were a lady of leisure, with the social graces and economic means that came with that status. Your body was proof. "To have a strong and muscular body is to be suspected of work, of service," wrote Dr. Dio Lewis in 1871's *Our Girls*, "while a frail, delicate *personnel* is a proof of position, of ladyhood."

While Lewis astutely noted this logic, that was not an endorsement of it. "It is true that many strong, muscular women are coarse and ignorant; they have given their lives to hard work, and have been denied all opportunities to cultivate their minds and manners," he wrote. "To compare such with the petted, pampered daughters of social and intellectual opportunity, and then to treat the strong body of the one as the source of the coarseness and ignorance within, and, in the other case, to treat the weak, delicate body as the source of the fine culture, is to reason like an idiot."

If you were one of those petted, pampered daughters who looked around and saw only other frail women, that's what you would consider the ideal. "The people we're around and the media we consume become our benchmark and measuring tape that we start to consider," says Linda Lin, psychotherapist and professor of psychology at Emmanuel College. "They're a picture of what's considered normal and desirable."

In *Lift*, a book on fitness history, author Daniel Kunitz recalls his own experience with the evolution of what he finds desirable. "Women with muscles were virtually nonexistent in my world, and so I associated anyone bigger than a bread stick with slovenly corpulence," he writes. "It was only after being around high-performance women that their muscles came to stand for vitality, vibrancy, health, and therefore for beauty."

Beyond just who's around you, what's going on around you, in terms of current events, makes a difference, too. During World War II, strong, capable women ruled, since they had to keep everything humming at home while the men were away. Women like Pudgy Stockton and actress Katharine Hepburn—tall, angular, athletic, a little brash—represented the kind of gal who could get things done. (Hepburn, it's worth noting, loved to exercise and did her own stunts. She often swam in the ocean and was always playing tennis. Her first big role was, interestingly enough, as an Amazon in a Broadway play. Before her, sporty actresses weren't widely admired.)

Once the fellas returned, old-fashioned values came back in a big way. Men were men, and women were women, and the contrast between the two was important. Enter Marilyn Monroe, with her soft, hourglass shape creating that curvaceous, coquettish appearance that defined femininity at the time.

Today we're sitting smack-dab in the middle of fourth-wave feminism, where issues such as workplace harassment, equal pay for equal work, sexual assault, and rape culture are taking center stage. Women are raising their voices and saying, "Me too," discussing subjects that have long been swept under the rug. To match a more powerful presence, it follows that a more powerful physical look is gaining appreciation.

EVEN WITH GENERAL PRINCIPLES THAT help us understand why certain bodies steal the spotlight at certain times, there's not a foolproof rubric. If we consider that what's difficult is desirable, Davidsdottir's body should be universally praised, given how many hours of work have gone into it.

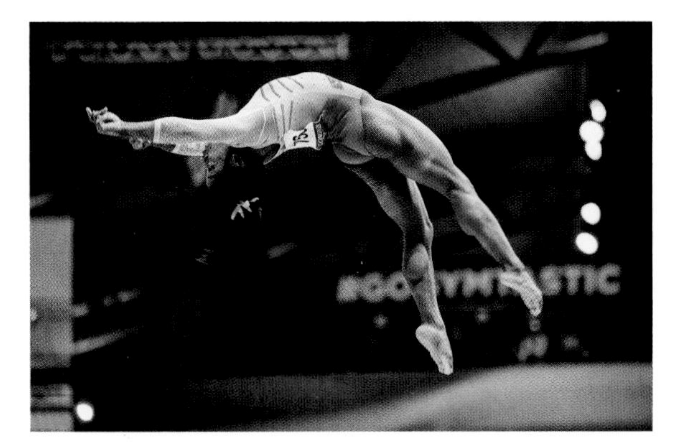

Simone Biles completes a balance beam routine in 2018. Although she was mocked for her muscles in her youth, they've helped her become arguably the greatest gymnast of all time.

"I know people think I am too muscular, or too big, or too thin, or too lean—there's always something," she told *ESPN* magazine. "But my body is the hard work that I've put into it, and I'm so proud of that."

Simone Biles, a gymnast widely considered to be the world's best, can relate. The enthusiastic teen burst into the hearts of casual gymnastics fans during the 2016 Olympics in Rio de Janeiro, winning over viewers with her giggly disposition, relatable crush on Zac Efron, and flawless routines . . . along with her ability to somehow stand head and shoulders above her competition even though she's only four-foot-eight.

While all gymnasts at this level are strong, with six-pack abs and substantial calves, Biles's muscular definition was next-level. This petite phenom was absolutely explosive. For her efforts, she took home a passel of gold medals, for individual all-around, vault, and floor, not to mention team gold and a balance-beam bronze.

Despite her obvious mastery of the sport, her success wasn't without controversy. Some interpreted Biles's muscles as inelegant and the incredible tricks she could perform with them as ungraceful. For Biles, this was nothing new. As a child, she worked hard in the gym, perfecting her handstands, back walkovers, and tuck jumps, and instead of admiring her dedication, some classmates sneered.

"I've learned to love my muscles a lot more than when I was younger, because I got made fun of a lot for them," she said in 2018. "People would say mean things at the time. They used to call me a 'swoldier,' which didn't make me feel the best. I wore sweaters or jackets all year long to cover my arms."

• • •

MANY WILL ARGUE THAT WOMEN with visible muscularity like Biles and Davidsdottir are simply unnatural. In this line of thinking, testosterone builds muscles, and testosterone is the domain of men. They have fifteen times more of it, after all.

But guess what? Women can build muscle at a similar rate to men. In fact, they may even build it faster. A recent meta-analysis of more than sixty studies looked at how the acquisition of strength between the sexes compared and found that overall, untrained men who started lifting got 29.41 percent stronger, while untrained women got 37.42 percent stronger.

Men still end up with more muscle in absolute terms because they start with more, but a well-designed training program will lead to comparable strength gains for women. If women's bodies weren't made to get stronger, why would their muscles respond to stimulus in much the same way as men's do? It's perfectly natural for women to gain muscle, and yet some still hesitate to reconcile that image with their picture of what a female should look like.

"For most of history, masculinity has been associated with strength and muscles, while femininity has been associated with frailty," says Lin, the psychotherapist who's studied body image. "They're polar opposites—the more in vogue muscularity is for men, the more in vogue frailty is for women."

These bodily standards are usually set by men, yet often they're reinforced by women. "Men get a lot of [flak] for ogling women's bodies. But when it comes to aesthetic standards, women are the enforcers," J. C. Herz writes in *Learning to Breathe Fire*, a book about the history of CrossFit. "Women are the ones who look at another woman's body and make negative remarks to her face, or communicate disapproval with a furrowed gaze or the curl of a lip. Women's bodies reflect a social order that's largely upheld by other women."

Take the example of actress Jessica Biel. In 2007, a photo of her popped up in the tabloids. She was on a beach in Hawaii, in a white bikini, playing a game. To a modern eye, she looks fit. She has some definition in her arms and lines on her abs. It's what you might describe as "toned." Lin says it was one of the first times she noticed a celebrity magazine showing a more muscular image of a woman in a positive light, communicating to readers that this was something to aspire to.

What's kind of mind-blowing is how Biel was perceived. In a 2009 survey conducted by trainer Leigh Peele, 36 percent of the two thousand women polled looked at this picture of her on the beach and said she was "bulky." A whopping 71 percent said they'd much rather appear too thin than too muscular or too fat. Additionally, more women at the time preferred to be "too fat" (18 percent) than "too muscular" (11 percent).

Peele offered this advice to readers: "Don't be afraid to be strong, if you want to be. Don't suppress what is inside of you because of what society dictates. No one else's judgment is worth questioning or abandoning your dream, and the more that people get used to seeing change, the faster change happens."

There's no doubt on that last point. You'd be hard-pressed today to find many people who think circa-2007 Biel is the definition of bulky. In just a decade's time, our outlook on muscularity has shifted. That's not to say we all desire lines around our abs, or that we necessarily should, but we have far more women in the public eye now who do lift heavy weights and sport more muscular physiques. The thought that femininity necessitates frailty is disappearing.

MANY MODERN WOMEN ARE REDEFINING what it means to look like an athlete in their given disciplines, perhaps none more famously than ballerina Misty Copeland. She was born with the perfect proportions to dance, but at nineteen, she found herself in an unfamiliar situation: her body was no longer the ballet ideal.

Until that point, her thin limbs, knees that sloped backward, small head, and big feet gave her all the tools for elegant dancing. But now, postpuberty, she was curvy and muscular. She was still the brilliant dancer she'd always been, but she was standing out for all the wrong reasons.

Copeland didn't start dancing until she was thirteen, practically geriatric in the world of ballet. And she was plucked from obscurity at a Boys' and Girls' Club, hardly the start for most stars on the rise, who first pad around in their pink tights and pint-size leotards about a decade earlier. But she overcame her lack of experience through sheer capability, and she soon had invitations for prestigious summer programs from all across the country. After summer stints at the San Francisco Ballet and the American Ballet Theatre in New York, she ended up in the ABT Studio Company, the highest rung on the training ladder.

Some felt she just didn't have the "look" to make that leap to professional dancer. Long, lithe, and white was the conventional expectation. Her frame was too muscular, her skin too black.

But Copeland's talent was undeniable, and she's used her gifts to change our perceptions of what a ballet dancer looks like. She ascended the ranks at the storied ABT to eventually become a principal dancer, the first African American woman in the company's seventy-five-year history to do so.

Even once she proved that she was the real deal, critics still used her body to denigrate her. "Though I have tremendous support from lots of people, there are so many others waiting to tear me down," she told the *Telegraph*. "There are people who say that I don't have the body to be a dancer, that my legs are too muscular, that I shouldn't even be wearing a tutu, that I just don't fit in."

To see her dance is to know that she was born to do this, and her muscles enhance, not detract from, the artistry she brings to the stage. Copeland knows this now, although accepting her womanly curves was difficult at first. She initially sought to punish her body, wishing it would return to its previous, childlike

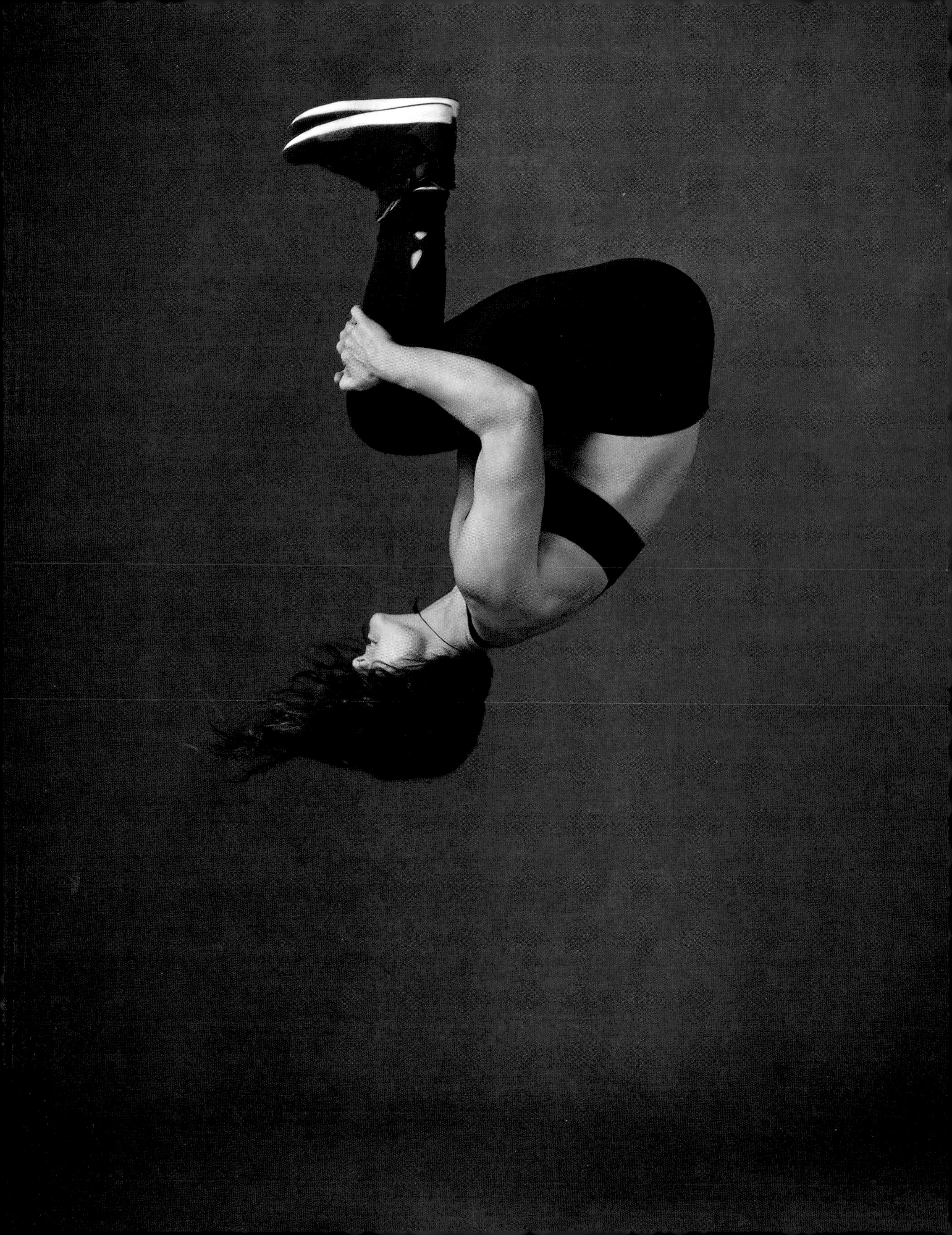

"I STARTED NOTICING MY LEGS WERE BIGGER THAN EVERYBODY ELSE'S AROUND THE SIXTH GRADE. OVER TIME, I FOUND OUT MY LEGS ARE WHAT GIVE ME MY POWER."

SYDNEY OLSON

FREERUNNER

---

form. But once she realized her body wasn't a fix-it project—and that she needed to take care of it, to make it as healthy as it could possibly be, even though it was different now—she began to dance with confidence and joy again.

What followed was one of the standout opportunities of her career at ABT, playing Firebird. For the iconic role, Copeland had to move her arms as if they were wings. As she practiced becoming birdlike over and over again, she developed a new type of muscle on her back. "It's pretty crazy to see the literal transformation of your muscles as you physically become a character," she wrote. "Your body actually transforms. As my back muscles grew, I felt my whole sense of self changing."

That muscle was functional and beautiful, even if it didn't look the way stodgy ballet purists might wish it did.

Being judged on looks is a topic Venus and Serena Williams could teach a master class on, given how often their muscularity and "otherness" have been used to disparage their talents. In 2001, radio sportscaster Sid Rosenberg said, "I can't even watch them play anymore. I find it disgusting. I find both of those, what do you want to call them—they're just too muscular." Fellow player Gabriela Sabatini suggested that they might "hit the ball too hard for the good of the game." Chris Evert likened them to Amazons, saying that women who didn't have their raw aggression struggled to compete with them. They've been described as pummeling, overwhelming, and overpowering by the media.

Then there's the Babe Didrikson treatment, where their womanhood is called into question. Anna Kournikova, considered one of the sport's most beautiful players of all time, reportedly said, "I hate my muscles. I'm not Venus Williams. I'm not Serena Williams. I'm feminine. I don't want to look like they do. I'm not masculine like they are." In 2014, the president of the Russian Tennis Federation called them "the Williams brothers." In what can only be interpreted as a direct shot at Serena, fellow player Agnieszka Radwanska's coach told the *New*

York Times in 2015, "It's our decision to keep her as the smallest player in the top 10. Because, first of all she's a woman, and she wants to be a woman."

The Williams sisters are also, in fact, women, and any attempt by others to tear down their bodies doesn't negate their accomplishments.

IT ISN'T EASY TO SHED the ideas that are ingrained in us from an early age about how we should look. Men are prized for doing, women for being. But it is something we can move past, and we might as well. Women's shapes vary an incredible amount, and we don't quite know why. Our bodies *can* be molded, as bodybuilders demonstrate, but only to a point. Letting go of what we expect them to be can be freeing, as Davidsdottir and Copeland discovered. Once you do, greatness might be just around the corner. Ultimately, a body is a vessel for living one's best life, not a showpiece to be benchmarked against the latest trend.

Plus, preferred body types come and go. Really, the only constant in the cultural norms of beauty is that they leave most women out. Tina Fey nailed it in her book *Bossypants*. "Now every girl is expected to have: Caucasian blue eyes, full Spanish lips, a classic button nose, hairless Asian skin with a California tan, a Jamaican dance hall ass, long Swedish legs, small Japanese feet, the abs of a lesbian gym owner, the hips of a nine-year-old boy, the arms of Michelle Obama, and doll tits."

That's a lot to live up to—in fact, impossible. But the one heartening aspect to the list is that it's probably more diverse than any standard from the past. Michelle Obama arms are worth flaunting now. Instead of communicating to the world that you're not a proper lady, a little bicep definition just says you can do push-ups.

On the subject of push-ups, Biles can do a whole lot of those, along with an arsenal of tricks made possible by her strong, muscular, swoldier-worthy arms. "I wish I could tell my younger self to be positive about my body," she said, "because when you learn to love your body, you learn to fall in love with yourself."

DANA TRIXIE FLYNN

YOGI

"Vulnerability is really letting people see your heart—that's the most beautiful strength."

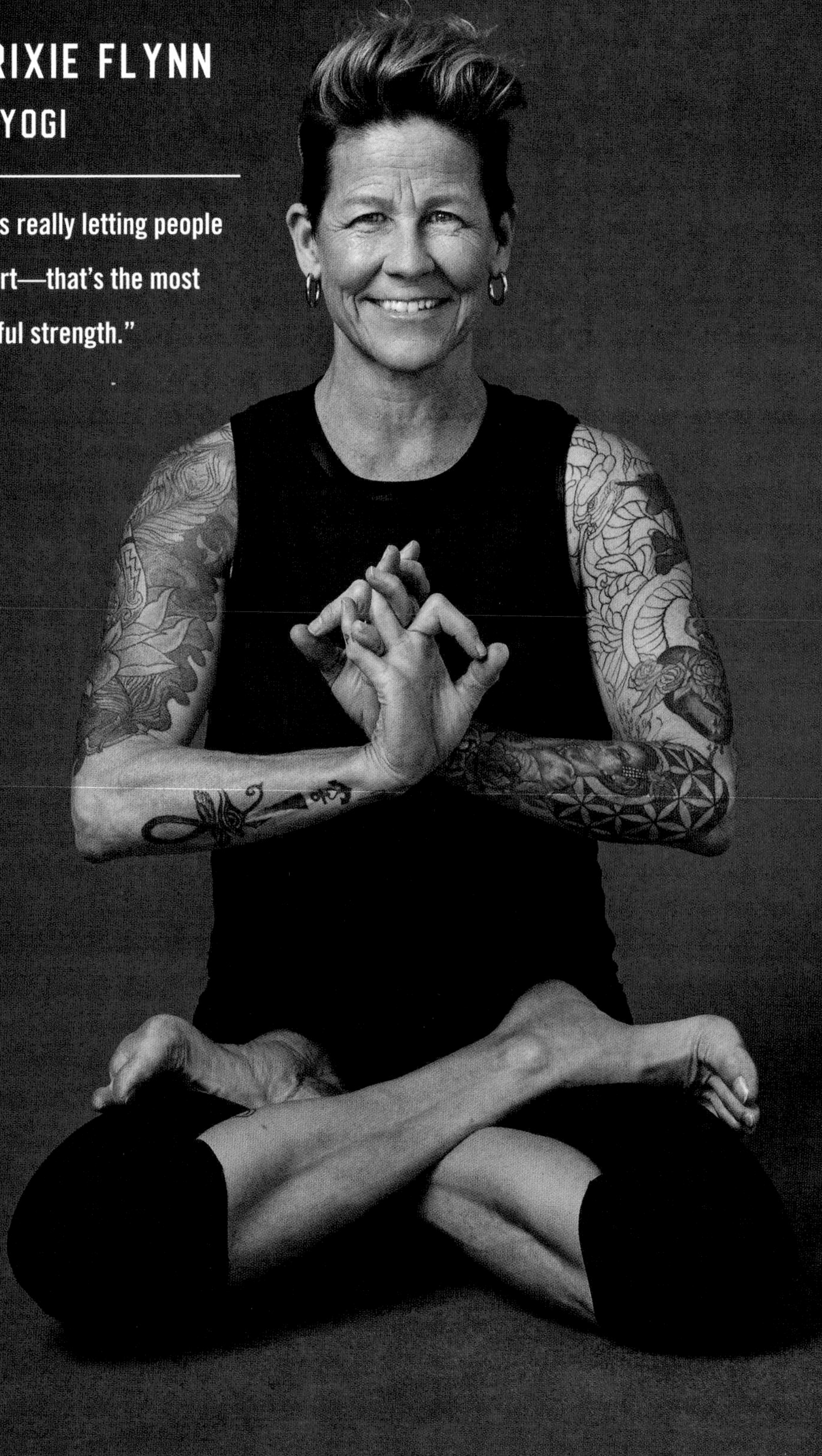

CHAPTER 11

THE POWER WITHIN:
HOW OUTER STRENGTH BREEDS INNER CONFIDENCE

Strength begets strength—and not just in the athletic sense. When women shed the cultural norms surrounding their appearance and pursue physical goals, they develop an incredible toolkit that serves them in all arenas of their life, well beyond the field, court, or gym.

"Confidence is where the page has turned: female strength so offended societal norms even a decade ago that picking up weights tended to cause anxiety in women," Daniel Kunitz writes in *Lift*. "Today resistance work is a means of building self-assurance."

IN 2002, LEI WANG'S LIFE was on a clear path. She was an MBA student at Wharton, one of the best business schools in the country, preparing for a high-powered career in the corporate world. She was exactly where she thought she should be.

A self-described book nerd, Wang loved to read because she had an insatiable curiosity about everything around her, so when her school organized a trip to climb Cotopaxi in Ecuador, she was in, even though the tallest "mountain" she'd ever climbed was a hill in Beijing.

Cotopaxi is an active volcano that stands 19,347 feet high. Its altitude can pose a significant challenge, but it's not considered particularly difficult from a technical perspective in the world of mountaineering, as long as one is fit—which, unfortunately, Wang was not.

"I went and it was totally a disaster," she says. "I came back throwing up, with a headache. I could only walk five steps and I needed a break."

Wang had assumed that since it was a school-related trip, it wouldn't be that strenuous, but that first attempt was so tough she found herself on her hands and knees, trying to inch forward. She realized she couldn't continue and would need to turn back. "At that point, I just slid down the hill," she says. "I couldn't even keep my legs straight."

She wasn't ready to give up just yet. Though she hadn't worked out at all prior to flying to Ecuador, now that she was there, she was determined to give it another try.

She rested for two days before attempting to summit once more, hoping the extra time would give her body a chance to adjust to the high altitude. Her goal was just to go as far as she could before turning around. This time, she made it to the top.

GROWING UP IN A POOR family in China during the Cultural Revolution, Lei Wang did not have sports on her radar. All she dreamed of was a career as a doctor or a scientist. After her successful Cotopaxi summit, she was satisfied. She'd quenched her curiosity and accomplished something difficult. She didn't think about mountaineering again until graduation, when a group of classmates organized a trip to Africa that included a jaunt up Mount Kilimanjaro.

Like Cotopaxi, 19,341-foot Kilimanjaro is considered suitable for beginners. Almost anyone with a good base level of physical fitness, who takes his or her time through the five climate zones so as to get properly acclimatized, can successfully summit. But Wang hadn't learned her lesson, and she wasn't any fitter this time than when she'd been in Ecuador.

"I was slow and weak," she says. "They let me take an assistant guide just for myself because everyone went at a faster pace."

She'd gone into the Cotopaxi adventure with complete ignorance, but she'd come to Kilimanjaro a little arrogant, and it slapped her in the face. "Kilimanjaro showed me how weak I was," she says. "I was not fast, I was not strong, I totally overestimated my fitness level. It made me worry about my health. I realized I'm in really bad shape and I'm still young—if I keep going like this, what's my life going to be?"

When Wang returned from the trip, she started jogging and doing yoga, and she signed up to run a half marathon as a motivational goal. Along her journey to get healthier, she saw the docudrama *Touching the Void,* a mountaineering survival tale, and says it woke her up. She realized that at the end of her life, she wouldn't be fulfilled by making a ton of money or being an exemplary employee. She needed something different, something that would put her body and mind into alignment. Now she was ready to get strong enough to climb another mountain—and this time, she would prepare.

Her goal was to get up Mount Everest, the vaunted pinnacle of all climbs, but she knew it would take time to work up to that level. So Wang decided to tackle the Seven Summits—the tallest mountain on each continent—and started with the easier ones first. She figured once she'd climbed the rest, she'd be ready for Everest.

While her former classmates were managing hedge funds and flying around the world for consulting gigs, she was scraping by, putting everything toward the new dream. A steady routine of hiking, running, rock climbing, and strength training got her ready for the task ahead, but the challenges mounted. On Denali, she was caught in a blizzard. On Vinson, she was struck with food poisoning. On Elbrus, she faced the very real risk of freezing to death. Making it to the top of Aconcagua took three attempts over a period of three years.

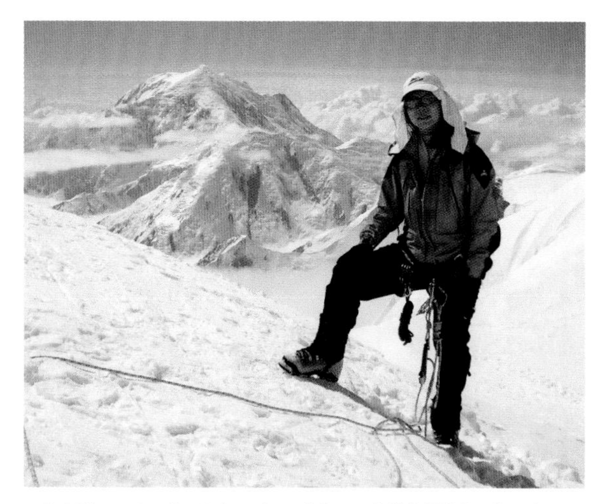

Lei Wang stands at the edge of Camp 3 (14,200 feet) on her way to the summit of Denali, North America's tallest peak.

Her mental resolve never wavered. Six years after setting her intention, she successfully summited Mount Everest, displaying the flag of Wharton at the top in homage to her beginnings. To her goal, she added skiing the North and South Poles, which together with the Seven Summits is known as the Explorers Grand Slam. Wang was the first Chinese woman and the first Asian American to achieve this distinction.

"You totally have a different perspective of who you are and what you are doing on the earth, what you are living life for," she says of reaching her goal. "You graduate from school, you get this job, and everyone else is doing the same thing. You compete with your colleagues to get a promotion, get more money, get a better title, and you don't even think about why you are doing it because everyone's doing it." Once she started climbing, Wang began to analyze why she was living her life the way she was, where her motivation truly came from, and what purpose her decisions served. "You get to see your own ability in a different perspective," she says. "You had no idea you were this strong."

THROUGH MOUNTAINEERING, WANG DISCOVERED THAT she wanted something different for her life from the conventional high achiever's path she'd been following. She gained the emotional strength to go against the grain, but if she'd truly wanted that corner office, her newfound physically strenuous hobby could have helped with that, too.

A 2013 global survey from Ernst & Young found that an overwhelming majority of women at the C-suite level in major companies had played sports growing up—a whopping 96 percent. The higher they were in their companies, the more likely they were to have played sports at a higher level. "Instead of just enjoying basketball and tennis and mountain climbing and skating for the sheer physical experience, women are starting to use the values and attitudes they have developed in these sports to get ahead in other areas," writes Sue Macy, who has authored several books on women's history and sports. "It turns out that loyalty, determination, competition, and teamwork are as important in government and the business world as they are on the athletic field."

Studies have also shown that girls who play sports are more likely to attend college, find a well-paying job, and work in male-dominated industries. (Just think of the players in the first intercollegiate basketball game, who went on to professions in areas such as academia and medicine that had historically been men-only.) Armed with the lessons from pushing their bodies, women can take bigger risks in their careers. They can set goals and systematically achieve them. And they can take pressure and turn it into performance.

WHEN LOOKING AT WHY THE majority of women throughout time haven't maximized their physical potential, we tend to blame the body. But the fault lies not so much in comparatively more fat mass on the legs or comparatively less muscle fiber in the arms but in those neurons firing away in the brain. Tell a girl early in life that she's not as strong as a boy, then keep reinforcing that message as she grows up, and you'll likely have the societal version of a self-fulfilling prophecy on your hands.

As humans, we are incredibly susceptible to the art of suggestion. The placebo effect has been proved time and time again. Whenever I feel a little congestion coming on, I pop a zinc tablet. It probably doesn't do anything, but I *feel* as if it does, and that may very well be more important than the small therapeutic effects.

When a woman has low expectations of herself, she achieves less. When she's told she has fifteen times less testosterone than a man and thus can't do what he can do, she won't try as hard. When she thinks she can't possibly be as strong as that guy a few feet away in the weight room, she's going to pick up smaller dumbbells than he's curling.

Conversely, if she believes she can achieve something, the odds of her doing so are much greater. In one study, fifteen male varsity athletes were given a four-month training program and told that the ones who made the most improvement would receive a course of steroids for the following month. Hoping to get some of that sweet, sweet (free, medically supervised) juice, the guys went for it. Six randomly selected participants were then given 10 milligrams a day of the performance enhancer Dianabol—or at least, that's what they thought. Instead, the pill was a placebo, but that didn't stop the gains train from rolling right on through. In three out of four of the exercises they'd been prescribed—bench press, squat, and military press—they improved by a total average of about 88 pounds. In the previous four months, when they were putting in the effort in order to be chosen for the steroid experimentation, they'd improved by about 17 pounds on average for the same three exercises.

Physiologically, nothing should have been different. But mentally, everything was.

A similar study took eleven national-level powerlifters and, five minutes before they maxed out on their three lifts—squat, bench press, and deadlift—gave them a pill they were told was a fast-acting steroid. It was actually saccharin. And oh, how sweet it was. The athletes beat their personal records by an average of 4 to 5 percent, which is a pretty big deal when you're already competing at a high level.

Then, for one week, they kept taking their saccharin "steroids" in preparation for testing their maxes again. Only this time, five of them were let in on the secret that it was all the equivalent of a handful of Skittles. Deflated by the news, when they went to lift, they all performed worse, some even sliding back to where they had started before the sugar pills, despite knowing they were fully capable of hitting those new PRs without steroid assistance.

Perhaps they were just tired from lifting a personal best relatively recently and a couple of tough training weeks? That sounds plausible, except that the six powerlifters who still thought they had a miracle drug on their hands mostly maintained their week-old PRs. A few even set new ones.

Everyone's body was capable of lifting more, but their minds weren't quite there. Tell a ten-year-old that the reason she can't do a pull-up is that she's a girl, and girls just don't have upper-body strength, and even if she *thinks* she's trying her hardest when she steps up to that bar and attempts to pull her chin over it, her mind might be putting up an obstacle she may never realize she needs to overcome.

These mental hurdles are everywhere. Canadian magazine *Best Health* started an article this way: "Ladies, if being able to do a pull-up is part of your fitness goals, it may just never happen, according to a new study."

Oh, really? What the study actually said was that after three months of training to strengthen their upper backs, lower their body fat, and improve their aerobic fitness, four of the seventeen women in the study could do a pull-up. Researchers thought it would be more. Some logical conclusions to draw from the study might be that pull-ups can be difficult or it may take longer than three months of training to master a pull-up. Telling women that no matter how hard they try, they'll never pull their chins above a bar—based on a study of a whopping seventeen people—is just rushing to confirm something we're already programmed to believe.

"Concluding that women can't do pull-ups has a more sinister effect," writes Kyle Hill, who's worked as a rock-climbing instructor. "I have trained many women who outright refuse to even try one. Women already believe that a pull-

“THERE REALLY IS NO FAILURE ONCE YOU’VE BEEN PLAYING FOR A CERTAIN AMOUNT OF TIME—EVERYTHING TURNS INTO LESSONS.”

JAZMYN JACKSON

SOFTBALL PLAYER

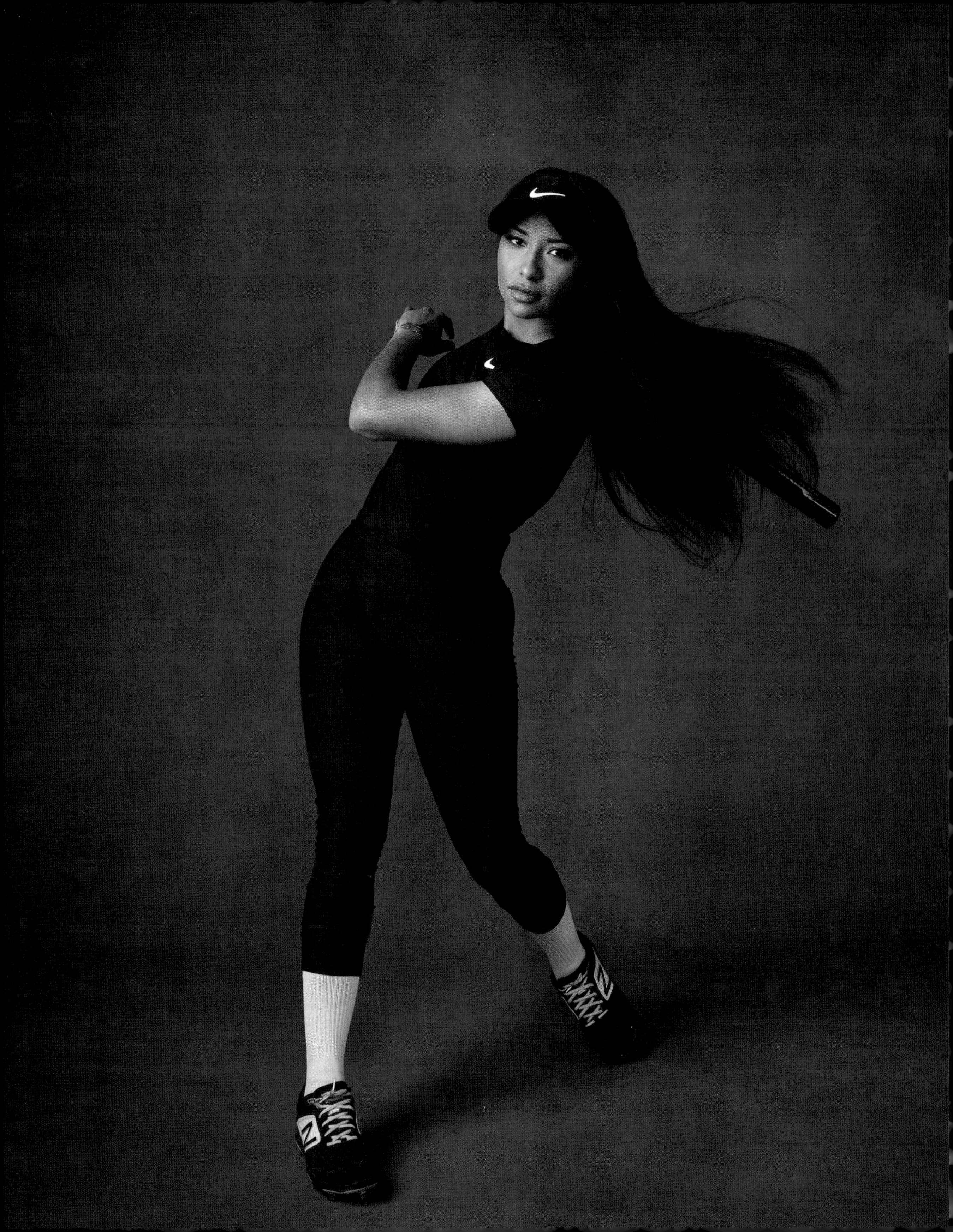

up is out of reach before their hands touch the bar. How many able women are discriminated against by this cultural truism?

"Peeling back the bias, to me it's obvious: if a woman isn't culturally dissuaded from trying, she is absolutely able to pull up and hit her head against the glass ceiling, smashing through it."

WHETHER WE'RE AWARE OF IT or not, there's always that cultural programming running in the background that for so long has told women that certain things aren't for them: muscles, lifting, heavy exertion. And yet those things have always been for everyone. Just think of the Scythians and their contemporaries—there were also Amazon-like figures in ancient Persia, Egypt, India, and China—confidently using their bows and arrows and muscled shoulders to ward off enemies.

Women, then, have been warriors for a long, long time, but they don't always see themselves that way. Growing up, Liefia Ingalls didn't play any sports. She thought of herself as a nerd, and that was the tiny box she occupied. In that box, there was no space for getting strong. "I pretty much considered that for other people," she says. "I thought, 'That's not a skill set of mine.' I didn't even really consider lifting or performing something I was worthy of."

She lifted weights casually in high school, primarily as a way to try to get skinnier. Her goals weren't performance-related, and she didn't push the boundaries of her strength. It wasn't until after college that she really focused on developing her physical prowess. "I started doing it for the enjoyment of lifting and the way it felt to become really strong," she says. "When that changed, that accelerated everything else."

She accelerated straight into competitions for strongman, a sport that involves picking up odd objects and moving them. This might mean pressing a log, carrying an atlas stone as far as possible, flipping a tire, or deadlifting a car. "I was always kind of attracted to the extreme stuff," Ingalls says. "I always had a challenge mentality where something is more interesting to me the harder it is. I want to try the thing that seems the most unreasonable."

For many people, strongman does look pretty unreasonable. Most of us don't lift cars unless a real emergency situation is going down and adrenaline is coursing through our veins. But Ingalls quickly realized she loved it—and was exceptionally good at it. The first time a major professional strongman competition was staged for women—the Arnold Pro Strongwoman in 2017—Ingalls was there. She wasn't a favorite to win, particularly given that there were no divisions based on size, and she was one of the smaller participants, but she had come to throw down.

After two days of competition that involved carrying kegs that weighed more than 200 pounds, hoisting a giant hammer in the air, and picking up ten concrete stones as fast as possible, Ingalls sat in second place going into the final day. In the penultimate challenge, competitors were tasked with one-hand pressing a 125-pound big-top circus dumbbell (this kind of dumbbell has globes at each end that are bigger than an adult human's head) as many times as possible in one minute. Eight presses later, her ponytail swinging back and forth as she used textbook technique, Ingalls had the event win. That vaulted her into first position as she prepared for the 500-pound axle car-tire deadlift (the axle bar had a diameter of two inches with no flex in it, much more difficult to grip than a traditional barbell). Picking it up and putting it down six times was enough to keep her in first place overall.

In front of a standing-room-only crowd, she accepted her prize of five thousand dollars and the Katie Sandwina Trophy, in honor of one of the original strongwomen.

"It was really validating," Ingalls says. "All that time and effort and energy and work I'd done paid off." You couldn't have convinced sixteen-year-old Liefia of this, but strength was for her, after all. "There's a disconnect in most people's goal-setting and achievement process," she says. "You just assume that if you can't do something, it's not for you. In reality, everything's for you if you're willing to put in the time and effort to learn and progress."

Through her strength journey, she's gained much more than muscle tone and the Katie Sandwina Trophy (although that is pretty dope, custom-made of solid bronze). She now runs her own strength-training business and imparts her wisdom to others. "The biggest benefit is the confidence in myself—that really came from acquiring physical strength and learning the process of lifting," she says. "It taught me I can do things that seem impossible; it led me to start my own business. There's been tons of failure and doubt, and myself from the past would've encountered those obstacles and given up. Now, it's 'How else can I approach this problem?' "

OUR BRAINS WILL ALWAYS TELL us we've reached our limits before that's truly the case. Studies show that this happens physically, mentally, and emotionally. That's understandable, given that our brains just want us to survive. They're not quite as concerned about whether we're fully maximizing our potential; they'd prefer us to have the cushiest life possible (which is kind of sweet, when you think about it). But we can train our brains to get comfortable with being uncomfortable, and one of the best ways to do that is to challenge our physical limits. When you don't think you can take one more step—and somehow, like Wang, you do—that's when you're really working on all aspects of becoming stronger.

We can't necessarily plot types of strength on an x and a y axis and draw an upwardly sloping line. The day you deadlift twice your body weight, you might not be ready to ask your boss for a well-deserved raise. Then again, you just might.

Yes, it's amazing to scale tall peaks and pick 500 pounds off the ground, but the life-changing magic comes from what you learn while pursuing these goals. As women discover their physical power, it opens doors in their careers and elsewhere. They might work up the motivation to try for a position they never thought possible or start a company that involves making a dream job of their creation, as

Ingalls did. They may even realize that a certain career no longer suits them. Wang now spends more days in the mountains than not and shares her story with groups instead of heading up a corporate team. She's happier than ever. "I have the freedom to do what I want to do," she says. "I can accomplish what I want to accomplish."

The meme "Carry yourself with the confidence of a mediocre white man" has taken off in recent years, and for good reason: it resonates. Not because white men are just bumbling along aimlessly, by any means, but because they are less prone to worry about being perfect. They're more likely to believe that when they're dropped into an unfamiliar situation, they'll find a way to succeed. A man will apply for a job if he has 60 percent of the listed requirements, while a woman won't apply unless she meets 100 percent of them, according to a Hewlett-Packard internal report. Pro obstacle-course racer Nicole Mericle has seen a similar effect in her sport. "There are more men participating, especially in the elite field—even though a lot of these men don't belong in the elite waves," she says. "I think this comes down to confidence. Men are overconfident and women lack confidence. If you're thinking about signing up, go for it! You're probably better than you think you are. Even if you do fail obstacles, don't worry—everyone fails things. There's no shame in trying something again."

When a woman takes the time to build her strength, she learns that failure is normal and that it can lead to incredible breakthroughs. "When something seems too hard or even impossible, you can look back and think, 'I had a similar impossible goal before and did it—why do I have to say no to myself this time?' " Wang says.

As the placebo studies demonstrate—and as the ancient Greeks knew—the mind and the body are inextricably intertwined. Strengthening one serves to reinforce the other. Only after Wang and Ingalls saw their bodies as strong did they realize that they possessed the inner strength to reach any goal they set. Maybe not today, but with an ample dose of confidence and resilience, there's always tomorrow.

SANDRIANA SHIPMAN

FLAT-TRACK MOTORCYCLE RACER

"I've always raced with the boys and never thought anything of it."

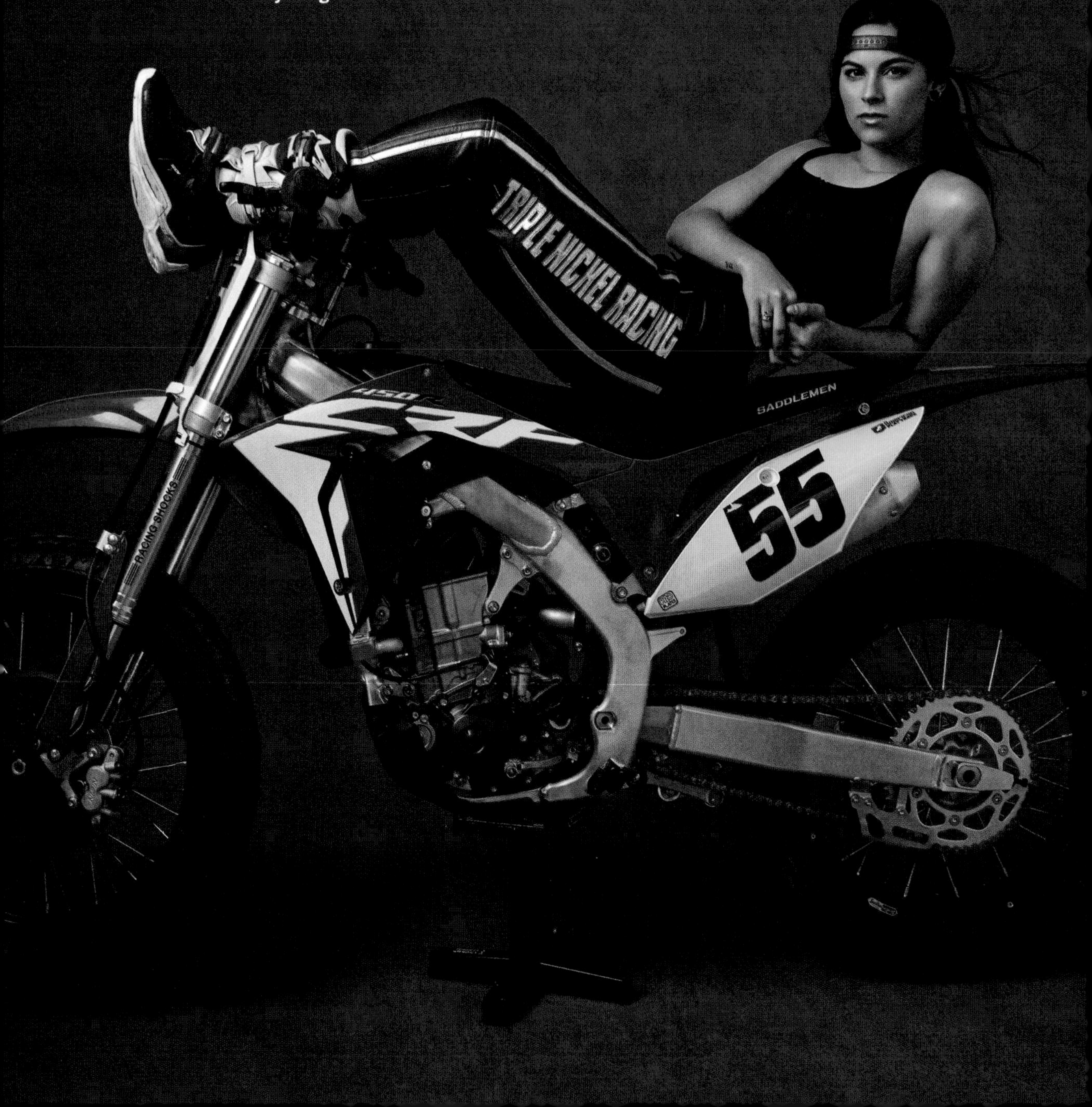

CHAPTER 12

STRONG(H)ER THAN YESTERDAY:

THE MODERN ATHLETE AND THE FIGHT FOR EQUALITY

Beginning in the 1970s, Billie Jean King championed equal opportunity to play in tournaments and equal prize money for men and women in professional tennis. "Everyone thinks women should be thrilled when we get crumbs," she said in 2016, "and I want women to have the cake, the icing, and the cherry on top, too."

Today's women realize that crumbs, however earnestly offered, really aren't enough. After winning the World Cup in 2015, the U.S. women's soccer team received a bonus of $1.725 million from the United States Soccer Federation—a seemingly big number, until you compare it with the bonus the men's team got the year before, when they *failed* to make it out of the Round of 16. For that, they earned an extra $5.375 million. Beyond the money, the women's team has long been shafted in other areas of compensation, such as travel, benefits, training, coaching, and medical treatment. In March 2019, the team sued U.S. Soccer, alleging that institutionalized gender discrimination has led to compensation that isn't equitable.

In between advocating for themselves, the players continued to improve their game. When the 2019 World Cup in France rolled around, they did even more to prove they deserved treatment on par with the men's team, winning most of their matches in triumphant fashion and capturing the title yet again. And still, criticism came. Was it polite to rack up thirteen goals against Thailand and then celebrate those goals? The players were called classless, uncivil, and patronizing by onlookers. Team captain Carli Lloyd explained that on the sport's biggest stage, in the most important tournament, you have to keep the throttle down at all times to maintain a winning mindset. This wasn't a youth soccer game played between two mismatched teams on a Tuesday night at the local high school field.

And then there were arguments about whether star players such as Alex Morgan and Megan Rapinoe celebrated their goals too much. After Morgan mimed sipping tea following her goal against England—a nod, she said, to the phrase "spilling the tea," which means to dish the truth—she was called disrespectful and distasteful by commentators. Morgan was surprised by the backlash, especially given how much more, shall we say, *boisterous* some men's goal celebrations can be.

"There is some sort of double standard for females in sports to feel like we have to be humble in our successes and have to celebrate, but not too much, and have to do something, but it always has to be in a limited fashion," Morgan said. "You see men celebrating all around the world in big tournaments, you know, grabbing their sacks or whatever it is."

Boys will be boys, but girls will be humble. Or at least that's how it's supposed to go, in many minds.

After the U.S. won the title game against the Netherlands, fans began to chant, "Equal pay!" The team returned to the United States to great fanfare, but still, no revised paycheck. "It's just been true that we'll never achieve, as women, any type of social equality without financial equality," said forward Christen Press after negotiations between U.S. Soccer and the players broke down in August, postvictory. "And we're looking for equal pay—not [just] talking about it any longer."

In the midst of the women dominating on the world stage, getting criticized for their unladylike celebrating, and continuing to battle for compensation they feel is rightfully theirs, something incredibly interesting happened: boys started to wear the jerseys of their favorite female players.

Columnist Heidi Stevens wrote in the *Chicago Tribune* about her fifth-grade son telling a story about multiple kids wearing Alex Morgan jerseys to school (conversation-worthy because he had a friend named Morgan, and they liked to joke that the jerseys were in honor of her).

"Wait, boys wear Alex Morgan jerseys?" Stevens asked her son.

"Yeah," he said. "Why?"

For a boy to be a fan of a female athlete, enough to sport her name on his back, is now cool for the youngest among us, but that's been true for a surprisingly short amount of time.

The national women's soccer team may be discouraged that the fight for fair pay doesn't look to be ending without at least a few more battles, but the players can feel heartened knowing that the next generation sees them with equality.

"The fact that fifth-grade boys and high school boys and, really, any age boys look up to women athletes in that way? To me, that feels like tremendous progress," Stevens wrote. "To me, that feels like we're getting somewhere."

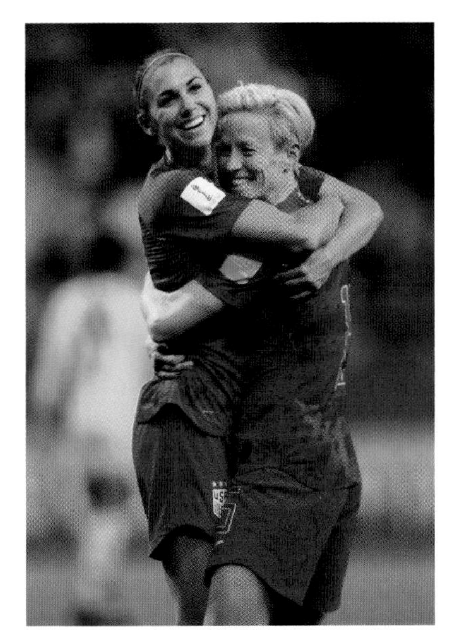

U.S. women's soccer players Alex Morgan and Megan Rapinoe celebrate during the 2019 Women's World Cup in France.

WE'VE STILL GOT ROOM TO improve. Female athletes today get 2 percent of airtime on *SportsCenter*, ESPN's flagship program, and not even half a percent of sponsorship money. That's a big deal for some athletes, such as track and field competitors, whose pay primarily comes from exclusive deals with companies. In May 2019, sprinter Allyson Felix, one of the most decorated athletes of all time, spoke out on her battles with sponsorship after getting pregnant. Nike wanted to pay her 70 percent less than she previously made, despite her being one of their most heavily marketed athletes. She accepted that, but when she asked for a contractual guarantee that she wouldn't be punished for taking the time to get back to fighting form after delivery, Nike refused. "It's one example of a sports industry where the rules are still mostly made for and by men," she wrote.

Long-distance runner Kara Goucher had her pay completely cut off while she was pregnant, although Nike didn't hesitate to announce her pregnancy in the *New York Times* for Mother's Day. All four Nike execs who negotiate sponsorships for track and field athletes are men.

Shortly after speaking out, Felix signed a clothing sponsorship deal with Athleta, which promised "full protection during maternity" and embraced her many roles, as an athlete, an activist, and a mother. In August 2019, Nike agreed to amend its contracts going forward, guaranteeing that a pregnant athlete's pay is protected for eighteen months, starting eight months before her due date.

Sometimes it can feel like two steps forward, one step back. There are actually fewer covers of *Sports Illustrated* with women on them today than there were thirty years ago (and that includes the swimsuit issues), and yet young athletes often don't realize that in the not-so-distant past, sports weren't so acceptable for girls to play.

Knowing the history of the women who have come before puts everything into perspective, and it keeps us aiming for equality in the areas, such as paychecks and publicity, where it's still lacking. "Some strong and angry women in my generation brought down some very big barriers for women in sports," said Dr. Karyn Marshall, the weightlifter, in a TEDx Talk. "We fought for it. Today's women are complacent, more entitled than insistent—that's why we've stopped accelerating. We're stronger than ever. We need to get angry again, we need to fight again."

IT'S IMPORTANT TO IDENTIFY HOW we can improve, but it's just as important to celebrate how many amazing women are killing it right now. In all of history, this is quite possibly the best time to be a strong woman, and equality is winning in plenty of places.

In the CrossFit Games, the top men and women earn the exact same prize money and get the same media coverage. The events are typically identical, with just the weights changing.

In tennis, all four Grand Slam tournaments now offer equal prize money to both sexes, thanks in large part to the efforts of King.

And then there's the phenomenon of *American Ninja Warrior*, the spin-off of a Japanese contest called *Sasuke* that started back in 1997. Because *ANW* bridges the gap between competitive sport and reality television, it doesn't necessarily play by the same rules as traditional sports. One of the ways it's changing the game is in the realm of gender segregation—that is, there is none. Men and women take on the same course, facing all the same obstacles. The women like it that way.

"I really appreciate it because it pushes me, it challenges me," says Barclay Stockett, who's quickly vaulted herself into the top tier of the sport even though she stands just five feet tall. "I have to be faster or stronger or more explosive for some of the same obstacles that others, just because of their size, can get through without necessarily a whole lot of strength or talent. It makes me have to work harder and I love hard work. There are no negatives for me."

When Dwayne "The Rock" Johnson was putting together his competitive reality show, *The Titan Games*, which debuted in 2019, he similarly kept the play-

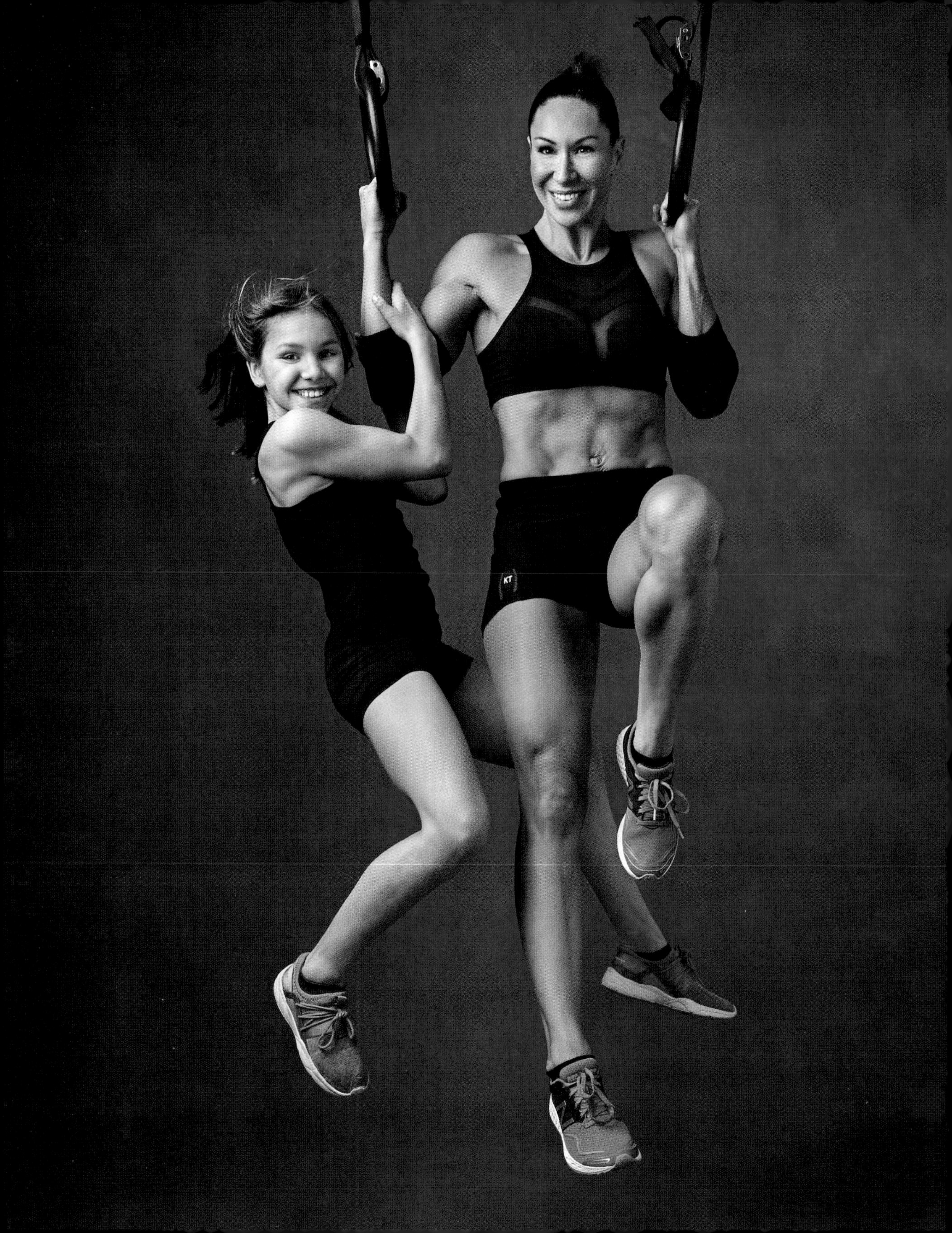

“WE’RE GOING TO LEAVE A LOT OF LEGACIES FOR OUR KIDS IN DIFFERENT WAYS, ABOVE AND BEYOND WHAT WE SAY. MOMS BEING HEALTHY AND ACTIVE IS A VERY POWERFUL THING FOR KIDS TO SEE.”

MAGGI THORNE

AMERICAN NINJA WARRIOR COMPETITOR

---

ing field the same for both sexes. "I did not alter my challenges for the women," he explained on Instagram. "If the men have to hammer through a 350-pound concrete ball, so do the women. If the men have to run through a 1,000-pound wall at Mount Olympus, so do the women. I have too much respect for women to change it, but more importantly—they wouldn't want it any other way. Because of this, the physical and mental arcs our women go through are simply spectacular and boundlessly inspiring. They got hurt. They bled. They conquered."

Keeping the obstacles the same puts these athletic feats into perspective. Only a few years ago, hardly anyone thought a woman could even make it up the Warped Wall, a signature obstacle from *ANW* that involves running up a steeply curved, 14.5-foot wall with a short runway. Now women are competing—and completing it—in record numbers. In the 2017 season, there were 20 percent more female applicants than the year before.

It may be a show created for entertainment purposes, but it's become so much more. One twenty-eight-year-old woman became a fan after battling anorexia for a decade, and the portrayal of powerful women transformed her life, as she detailed on Reddit:

> Something in my brain completely changed watching all of these amazingly strong and disciplined women compete. I wanted to be like them in every way—happy, healthy, strong. The more I watched, the more motivated I got, and I finally got the courage to go back to the gym and get into good shape.
>
> I'm not interested in how much I weigh, how many calories I'm burning, or what I look like in the mirror. I don't weigh myself because that's not my goal anymore. I'm in the gym 4–5 days a week lifting weights, doing leg press, using the rowing machine, swimming laps in the pool, etc., but I'm building muscle and loving it. I find myself rubbing

> my hands on my thighs or my arms feeling my muscles getting bigger and I can't get enough of it. I used to do this to try and feel my bones, or be able to wrap my hands around my thighs to prove how skinny I was. For the first time in my life, I feel like I am mentally capable of having a healthy relationship with exercise and leading a healthy lifestyle.

That is what happens when you give women a challenging set of physical obstacles and trust that they are capable of conquering them. They build a confidence in themselves that radiates and spreads to everyone around them, even people they will never meet.

EQUAL OPPORTUNITIES ARE IMPORTANT FOR the country's top athletes—such as the players on the U.S. women's soccer team and sprinter Felix—whose livelihoods depend on it. But it's not just the most elite athletes who benefit. When physical strength is a quality that's valued in everyone—boys and girls, men and women, nonbinary and gender-nonconforming folks—everyday athletes realize that their strength matters, too.

When a woman learns what her body can do—and how to appreciate it for its capabilities instead of scolding it for its faults—she feels more comfortable in her own skin. A three-time CrossFit Games winner and a 2016 Olympian in weightlifting, Australia's Tia-Clair Toomey has learned firsthand how powerful building physical strength can be. "I was so intimidated when I first started, but now I feel very confident walking into a room full of people I don't know, so it's changed my life," she says. "Now I'm living this dream for myself and realizing just how empowering it is."

If the area of strength sports is a medieval castle of masculinity, women are powering the battering ram, ready to knock down those sky-high gates. They're shooting fire arrows over the walls. They're climbing ladders and finding windows to get in.

Between 2015 and 2016, the number of female powerlifters doubled, the biggest increase in the history of the sport. Women now make up a third of participants. In March 2019, Stefi Cohen passed the five-plate milestone—that's five 45-pound plates on each side of the barbell—when she squatted 495 pounds, more than any man or woman has ever done before in the 123-pound weight class. In Olympic weightlifting, female participation rose 125 percent from 2012 to 2016, and women's world records have crept up to around 80 percent of those set by men.

University of Texas assistant professor of instruction Kim Beckwith, who began powerlifting in the late 1980s under Jan Todd and now helps coach the team at UT, has seen the sport evolve over the years. "It's really a personal adventure to improve your own abilities," she says. "For women, it gives them a certain element of freedom that they now accept is their right. They're not restricted; they can do anything."

For many, it's surprising to find out just how strong they are. For hundreds of years, women have been told that weakness is sexy. Men are supposed to be big and powerful. Women are dainty and beautiful. Blur those lines, and you just might be a man-hater, ugly, misguided, or all of the above. Until *bulky* is no longer the scariest descriptor that can be used in reference to a woman's body, we won't know what's truly possible.

We are getting closer to finding out, though. Like the Spartans, we recognize that it doesn't make sense to limit strength to the male of the species. And we've got more reasons than our ancient ancestors did to encourage women to lift. Beyond building an overall healthier society, we understand that strength confers mental and emotional benefits. That it creates social change. That it saves lives.

STRONG WOMEN ARE HERE TO STAY. They exist everywhere you turn, from television to social media to your own community. They are more sure of themselves than ever before, less willing to let society's standards for how they should look and talk and act detract from the way they harness their power.

U.S. soccer forward Megan Rapinoe is a lightning rod for these issues: female, muscular, outspoken, gay, unapologetic. Like the circus stars of a century ago, she's here to use her platform for the greater good, whether that's continuing to speak out on equal pay for women or taking a knee during the national anthem to advance the conversation on racial equality in the country.

"Putting yourself out there is hard, but it's so worth it," Rapinoe said in 2016. "I don't think anyone who has ever spoken out, or stood up or had a brave moment, has regretted it. It's empowering and confidence-building and inspiring. Not only to other people, but to yourself."

It is largely because of the long line of women who have come before today's stars that they're able to do what they do, to be celebrated as athletes while simultaneously advocating for more opportunity, more respect, more equality.

Every woman along the way who's picked up a barbell, sprinted as fast as she could, or played ball with the boys has contributed to this rich legacy. History books may gloss over the role that physical strength plays in a woman's life, but it's clear that we'd be in a very different place without it, a place of less confidence, more fragility. A place of doubt that's not followed up by knowing one can overcome. A place where the weaker sex is all women could ever expect to be. A place where boys don't wear the jerseys of their favorite female players.

But now they do. They want to be strong like her.

ALICIA ARCHER

FLEXIBILITY ENTHUSIAST

"The body is incredible when you give it a chance to learn something new."

AFTERWORD

I was working on this book when I had the opportunity to travel to Iceland and participate in the Spartan Ultra World Championship. Most of the athletes there were racing for twenty-four hours, but having no training in either obstacle-course racing or ultramarathons, I signed up for the "sprint" course, a nearly seven-mile loop over unforgiving terrain that included carrying buckets of gravel long distances, sliding down sheets of ice, traversing monkey bars, climbing ropes, hoisting giant sandbags, and much more that I've mostly blocked from my memory.

Before the race, Spartan founder Joe De Sena explained that he had designed the course to be as difficult as logistics could reasonably support. When he was trying to identify the ideal location for the race, Iceland in December came to mind. "My team came back and said, 'No, because there's no light and it's extremely cold,'" he told me. "And I said, 'Perfect.'"

His team was not mistaken. The conditions were harsh. But Iceland was also incredibly beautiful in the way that only stark landscapes can be. When I crossed the finish line, I had such an immense gratitude for my body and an appreciation for myself that I have made it a priority to stay strong so that I can do things like fly to Iceland on only a few days' notice and complete bonkers obstacle courses. I wasn't the best, by any means, but without any special training, I did it. My glutes and biceps and quads and abdominals and whatever muscles are in my forearms showed up for me.

Being strong makes life easier and more fun. Because fun is what I had out there on that obstacle course, even if it didn't exactly feel that way when my life flashed before my eyes as a fellow competitor slid uncontrollably down a sheet of ice, narrowly avoiding launching me off the mountain as I swiftly jumped out of the way. "You're really lucky you have quick reflexes," he told me, still dazed.

I am lucky to have quick reflexes—although I like to think there was a little skill involved, too—but I'm even more lucky that I grew up when I did, after a lot of hard work by female athletes had been accomplished that helped make it possible for me to compete in a race of this kind.

Growing up, I played whatever sport I wanted, without much fear of being considered masculine, which might be why I was so surprised at the reaction when I announced that I planned to enter a bodybuilding contest. My fit fam was excited, wanting to know the details about my training plan and the color of my sparkly bikini. My actual family, on the other hand, was mostly in disbelief.

"Why are you hanging out with those disgusting women?" a relative asked after seeing a photo on social media of me supporting some of my bodybuilding teammates at a show.

"Disgusting" is a harsh word to describe anyone, and yet people who would never refer to someone who is obese or alarmingly thin or even slovenly as disgusting have no problem hurling that label at women with above-average muscle definition. Building strength seems to be an invitation for body commentary and even touching. While I was in training, a few well-meaning women asked if they could feel my muscles, a request that caught me off guard.

"Women are pigeonholed into such pressure to look a certain way, it's unreal," says Steve Wennerstrom, the women's bodybuilding historian. "It's something I've seen since I was young enough to understand what kind of pressure that is. When you step outside of that kind of paradigm, you're in trouble—you're going to be criticized or dealing with the negativity."

I expected people to be curious—it was certainly different from my typical fitness pursuits—but the disdain was perplexing. When I visited home a few weeks before my show, the commentary shifted from the people I was keeping company with . . . to me. "You look like a man!" another relative exclaimed. I think it was meant to be a joke, but considering that I still had plenty of fat, at least by bodybuilding standards, stored in those female strongholds of the hips, thighs, and chest, objectively this just wasn't true. But even if I had been leaner or more cut or as flat as a pancake, that wouldn't have made me any "manlier." And I was pretty lucky, as far as the comments went. Like Sandwina's a century before me, my muscular definition fit into one of the contemporary standards of an ideal body—in this case, a low-body-fat version of an hourglass shape—and this inoculated me from reactions that could have been much worse.

I was also amazed by how very worried everyone became about my romantic prospects. One of the most frequently asked questions I received was, "But how will you date?" Others would say things like, "Wow, look at you! Guys must love your muscles!" or "Don't get too strong. Men don't find that attractive." They're opposite sentiments, but the common thread running through the commentary was how bodybuilding was affecting my relationship with men.

When I signed on the dotted line to start training for a competition (yes, there was an actual contract involved), how men would perceive me wasn't a consideration. I didn't do it to be more sexually attractive, and I didn't think it would make me more or less likely to find a significant other. It simply didn't factor into my decision-making process, and I wish society at large didn't feel the need to frame women's fitness decisions in the context of how they affect their marriage or child-rearing prospects. We have come so very far, and yet our definitions of womanhood remain somewhat constrained by what a person should look like—and if she doesn't look that way, she must make up for it by wearing bows in her hair or talking about her children or snagging a guy. (Even the incomparable Babe

Didrikson Zaharias felt the need to defend her femininity in her autobiography by saying, "I was always interested in the women's things around the house, like cooking and sewing and decorating. I loved all the pretty things, and I still love all the pretty things.")

I struggled with these ideas while training for my show. In the end, I went onstage with five-inch heels, hair extensions, glittering jewelry, false eyelashes, and fake nails, and I smiled and strutted—or tried to, at least—and attempted to attract the judges' attention my way. It was so different from who I normally am, and I liked it for that reason. I felt like an actor taking on a role. I also disliked it for that reason. Was playing up an expression of traditionally defined femininity undermining the message I wanted to convey? Were my actions saying, "Hey, a little muscular definition is OK if you still look good in a swimsuit that's small enough to fit into a sandwich-size Tupperware container"?

For me, bodybuilding was a goal that fell into the same category as many other things I've done in recent years, including running a marathon, completing a triathlon, summiting a 14,000-foot mountain, and riding a bike 206 miles. It was hard work, and I did it to prove that I could. I wanted both to be strong and to look strong, regardless of what others thought. I know that I'm still influenced by society's definition of what is attractive, and I can't pretend that the positive comments I received about my appearance while I was training didn't please me on some level. (Sprinkled in with the criticisms, of course, as noted above.) But I can honestly say that what touched me the most was when my mom's cousin, who'd been following my journey unbeknownst to me, showed up to cheer me on. I later found out she was inspired to get into the gym and work toward a pull-up. I felt just a tiny shred of what Pudgy Stockton must have experienced when she got all those letters from women who saw her and felt moved, quite literally, to improve their health and well-being.

• • •

MY MOM'S COUSIN MAY HAVE found some inspiration in me, but I found a huge dose of inspiration on my way back from the Spartan Ultra World Championship, on a layover in Chicago. I struck up a conversation with a man sitting near me. "You should meet my wife," he said. "She's very strong."

Fortunately, I got to do just that a few minutes later. Retired businesswoman Edie Edmundson recounted the story of how, at age seventy-five, she stood in the store, staring down a 25-pound bucket of kitty litter. There was a problem: she couldn't get it into her cart. "I asked a customer to take it down," she said. "I thought, 'This is ridiculous. I can't depend on other people to do simple things for me.' "

Now eighty-two, Edmundson says she was always active growing up and had been the captain of the drill team. But no one back then lifted weights, not even the boys. She never really considered it an activity she might like to try until that wave of frustration came over her in the grocery-store aisle.

In a case of serendipitous timing, she found her solution when she won a one-month membership to a CrossFit gym around that same time. They started her off with an assessment of what she could do. She remembers that she couldn't complete a single sit-up or get off the floor without using a box to pull herself up. She started a program of lifting light weights, and within a couple of weeks, she felt her strength returning. She was able to do sit-ups, and getting off the floor was becoming easier. A year in, she'd lost fat, gained muscle, and felt she looked better in her clothes, although that was just a fringe benefit. "I was starting to feel more energy," she told me. "I really liked being able to do the day-to-day things better, like pulling a suitcase through an airport and going up and down stairs."

Once she could lift 25 pounds, she went for 35, and then for 50. On her eighty-first birthday, she deadlifted 121 pounds, a fact that lit up her face to share. "The body is meant to work, and when it doesn't work, it gets really lazy," she said. "The more you sit, the more you want to sit."

As much as Edmundson understands the gravitational pull to want to sit (how lovely it is to curl up with a good book), it's worth it for her to keep moving. She takes no prescribed medication, her bloodwork levels are all perfectly normal, and she's found a great community through getting stronger. "I absolutely love working out with the people who are much younger than me," she said. "They treat me as an equal. They're so positive and encouraging. Even if you come in and you're kind of tired and you've had a busy, stressful day, it doesn't take long before you're smiling because your mind is concentrating. It's good mentally and good socially for me."

Edmundson can do all those things that younger people often take for granted—walk to the mailbox, stand on her feet to cook, and get out of a chair. And of course, that bucket of cat litter is no longer a problem. In fact, she now finds herself helping others in the grocery store.

It's one of my favorite stories from the dozens of amazing tales I've heard while working on this book. I guess it's because Edmundson is so normal. We all love to cheer for the U.S. women's soccer team and watch in awe as Simone Biles does gymnastics tricks no mere mortal has ever performed before, but their level of athletic talent is on another plane. Here is a woman in her eighties proving that you don't have to possess a superhuman-style capacity in order to benefit from pursuing strength-based goals—you just have to be willing to put in the effort. "I've had people who have said, 'You're my inspiration,' and I've said, 'Anybody can do this; it's just a mindset of getting yourself to the gym,' " Edmundson says. "I don't think I'm unusual; I think I'm normal. You're never too old to start."

MY GOAL IN HIGHLIGHTING STRONG women is not to say everyone *must* be like them but to say everyone should feel *able* to be like them. For so long, we've actually trained our bodies to be weak and inefficient to fit a cultural expectation. This only serves to make us not trust ourselves, to slump our shoulders and suck in our stomachs and doubt that we're capable of great things. I like the take of Molly Galbraith, cofounder and woman-in-charge of Girls Gone Strong, a resource for evidence-based health and fitness info. "I've evolved over time from really pushing the agenda of strength training to believing deeply in women's autonomy and right to choose what they get to do with their bodies," she says. "I do hope they strength train, because it's super awesome—it's incredibly beneficial for physical health and for building confidence and self-efficacy—but it's more important to me that they get to choose what they want."

I've made the conscious choice to work on getting stronger, and it's a choice that I value—and never take for granted. Thanks to Cynisca and Madame Anderson and Sandwina and Pudgy Stockton and Jan Todd and Misty Copeland and countless others who span the ages, I can continue to build my strength without concern that my uterus might fall out or that I'll never attract a man or that I'll just be wasting my time on a futile pursuit.

Unlike the real-life Amazons, I don't live a nomadic lifestyle where I need to be tough enough to defend myself. If I'm ever unearthed long after this life has passed, my bones won't show a traumatic existence of breaking and fusing back together over and over again. (For that, I am quite thankful.) But I like knowing that if I'm ever scrambling up the side of an Icelandic mountaintop again or transported to the steppes of Eurasia atop a horse, bow in one hand, spear at my side, I'll be strong enough to be just fine.

ATHLETE BIOS

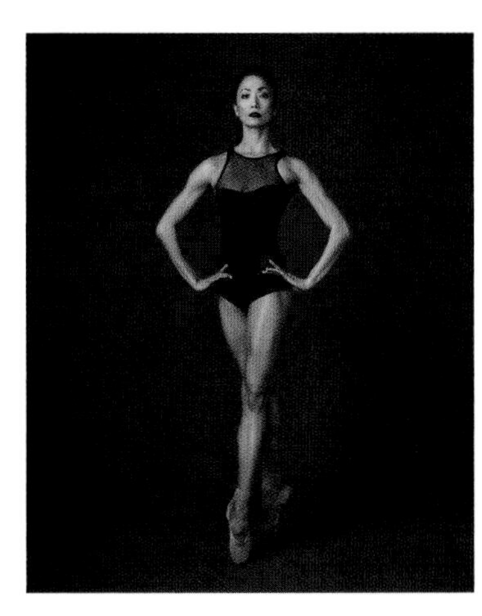

STELLA ABRERA

BALLET DANCER

BORN: 1978

HOMETOWN: South Pasadena, California

WHAT SHE'S KNOWN FOR: Abrera joined classical ballet company American Ballet Theatre, based in New York City, in 1996 as a member of the corps de ballet. In August 2015, she was appointed principal dancer, the first Filipina American in ABT's history to earn the coveted rank.

Stella Abrera was a pretty typical five-year-old watching cartoons when her eldest sister told her she was turning into a couch potato. While that criticism is debatable, something very good came out of the proclamation: Abrera's sister took her to a local dance studio, where she immediately fell in love with ballet. In a pre-YouTube world, her mom drove her to the library so she could check out dance videos and pore over them at home. By age twelve, she knew ballet was what she wanted to pursue as a career.

When Abrera was twenty-nine, she suffered a back injury that took her offstage for two years. "Up until that point, I didn't realize that one could not be invincible," she says. "It was an extremely challenging time, but I was determined to get back onstage. I just knew that I could. It was a painful, disappointing, and frustrating recovery process, but I was very stubborn in getting back."

To keep her body strong and prevent injuries, Abrera incorporates cross-training into her routine, including Gyrotonics, swimming, and working out at the gym. "What a dancer needs to do to keep his or her body in tip-top shape is a lot," she says. "I don't think people know how much goes into it."

That's by design. Abrera's job is to make the dancing look effortless, to transport the audience into another world. And in all her roles—some of her favorites include Juliet in *Romeo and Juliet*, Giselle in *Giselle*, and Gamzatti in *La Bayadère*—she does just that.

"I've always been driven to be a dancer," she says. "It was very simple. Whatever obstacle came my way, I did everything in my power to overcome it and dig deep and persevere."

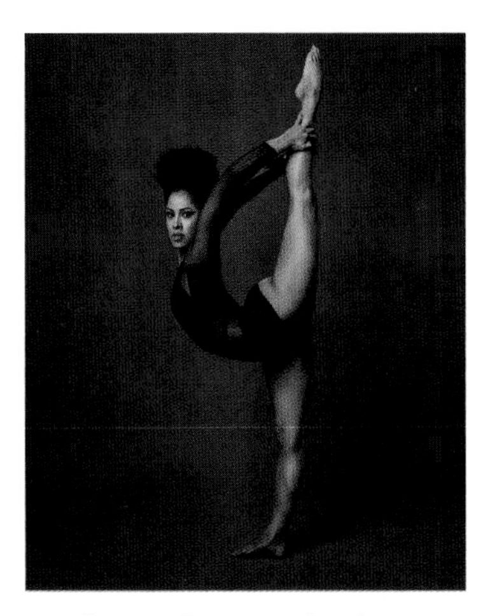

ALICIA ARCHER

FLEXIBILITY ENTHUSIAST

BORN: 1985

HOMETOWN: Bronx, New York

WHAT SHE'S KNOWN FOR: A specialist in bodyweight strength training and flexibility, Archer is an in-demand fitness instructor in New York.

Alicia Archer grew up dancing, learning the standard ballet, tap, and jazz routines that are performed at end-of-summer showcases. In high school, when she decided she wanted to pursue dance at the next level, she was disappointed to discover that she'd never learned the fundamentals most serious dancers had by her age. She started practicing ballet six days a week preparing to audition for the Ailey

School, connected to the Alvin Ailey American Dance Theater, a modern dance company in New York. Her work ethic paid off with an acceptance, but upon graduation, she had no offers to dance professionally. "No one wanted me," she says. "No one reached out to me and said they loved how I danced."

After getting a front-desk job at fitness club Equinox, Archer began taking group fitness classes. She'd always been intrigued by circus arts and slowly started working on skills such as flexibility, handstands, and balance, still wishing these were things she would have mastered in her youth but pushing past the frustration. "I would stay before and after class to practice and do a little more every day," she remembers. "There were times I wanted to take a nap, but I knew these little moments of training add up."

Eventually, she became a popular fitness instructor, and she now works to motivate and inspire others every day through her classes and on social media to become holistically healthy. "There's so much misinformation and misconception in the fitness industry right now about having to punish your body in order to get great results," she says. "I want to help people understand that function is far more important than aesthetics."

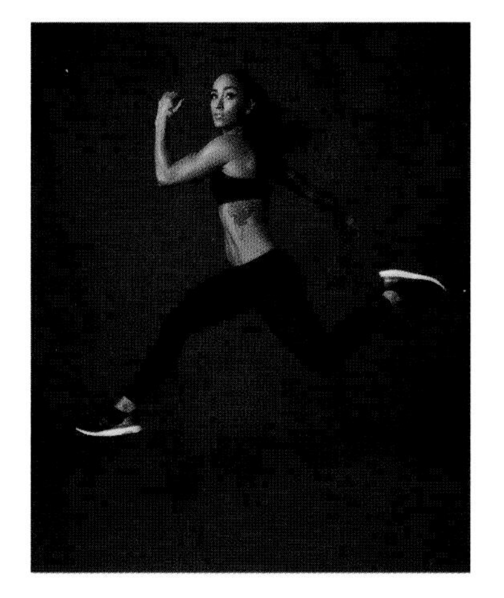

ROBIN ARZÓN

ULTRAMARATHONER

BORN: 1981

HOMETOWN: Philadelphia, Pennsylvania

WHAT SHE'S KNOWN FOR: Arzón is an ultramarathon runner and the best-selling author of *Shut Up and Run*. She is also the vice president of fitness programming for Peloton.

Today, Robin Arzón is known as a stylish ultramarathoner and always-inspiring Peloton instructor, but fitness was not woven into her DNA. No one in her family played sports, and growing up the daughter of a Cuban mother and a Puerto Rican father, she saw herself as the straight-A student, the arts-and-crafts kid, but never the athlete.

It was a traumatic experience during college that changed the trajectory of her life. Arzón was in a bar when a gunman stormed in and held everyone inside hostage. He doused the group in kerosene and chose Arzón as a human shield between him and the police. Eventually, he was attacked by a hostage and captured. After that, Arzón was determined to live each day as if it were her last. While in law school, she picked up a pair of running shoes and ran her first mile at the age of twenty-three—a way, she believes, of processing the pain that still lingered. With each step, she evolved into the athlete she never thought she could be. "It was through running where I really discovered my ability to transform and tell my own story," she says. "The inner confidence that comes from enduring a tough run is the most valuable thing that I've discovered."

After working as a corporate litigator for seven years, Arzón had a decision to make. Her passion for fitness was growing, and she could continue fitting it in around her schedule, or she could take the leap and turn it into a career. She left the law firm behind and fully embraced a self-created path that revolves around motivating others. "There's always an opportunity to level up, there's always an opportunity to be one percent better than yesterday," she says. "People who are constantly curious about their potential tend to work out."

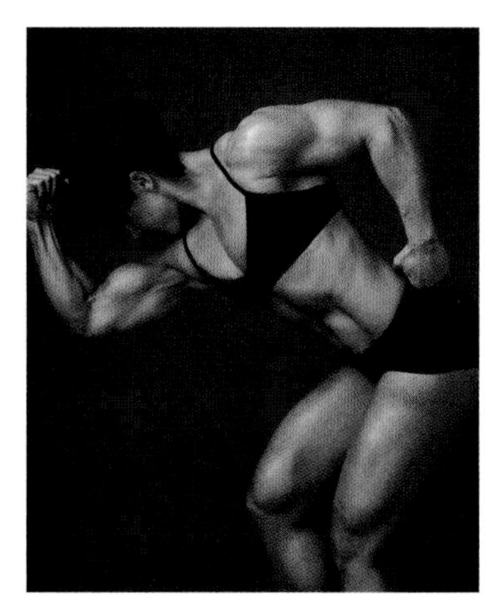

DANA LINN BAILEY

BODYBUILDER

BORN: 1983

HOMETOWN: Reading, Pennsylvania

WHAT SHE'S KNOWN FOR: Bailey became the first IFBB physique pro in history in 2011 and the first Ms. Physique Olympia in 2013. She owns a clothing line, a supplement company, and a gym.

A six-sport athlete in her youth who went on to play soccer at West Chester University, Dana Linn Bailey was always athletic. Once her final year of soccer was over, she needed a new fitness outlet, and that was when she found her way to lifting. Her then-boyfriend and now-husband, Rob, introduced her to the weight room. "I just followed exactly what he did," she says. "I was benching, I was deadlifting, I was squatting—I was just doing whatever the guys were doing. Little did he know he would create a little monster."

A little monster, indeed. DLB, as she's known by her fans, started competing in bodybuilding shows in the figure category in 2006, although she was often criticized by the judges for being too muscular. When the International Federation of Bodybuilding and Fitness (IFBB) announced the new physique division, a step up in muscularity from figure, Bailey was on the verge of leaving the sport, but this new category was her best shot to get a coveted pro card, the designation that separates amateurs from professionals. When the first show that would be handing out a pro card came around, she knew she had to enter. Low on funds, she did the entire prep herself, without the help of a coach to plan out her training or diet. She had to borrow a car to drive to the competition and haggle at the front desk of a hotel to find a place to sleep for a few hours.

The effort was all worth it when she came away with first place. "I spent so many years being last place and being told I was too muscular, too lean, too masculine, that I should change my hair, change the way I dress, be sexier," she says. "Throughout all the criticism, I somehow did not lose myself. Words still can't describe that feeling when I won."

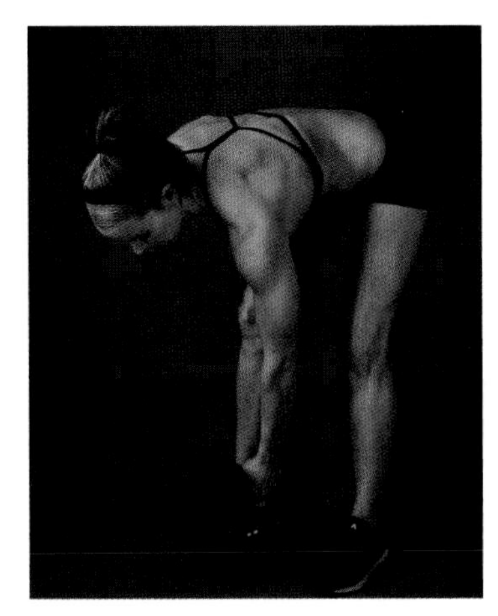

LINDY BARBER

CROSSFIT ATHLETE

BORN: 1989

HOMETOWN: Louisville, Kentucky

WHAT SHE'S KNOWN FOR: Barber competed in the CrossFit Games twice as an individual and three times as part of the storied Team CrossFit Mayhem Freedom. They won twice, including Barber's final year of competition in 2018.

There might not be a sport Lindy Barber hasn't tried. Volleyball, basketball, dance—she was even on a competitive jump-rope team for eight years. But in middle school, when it was time to pick a main sport, it was soccer where she decided to focus her efforts, going on to play for two years on the varsity team at the University of Dayton.

When that was through, she missed being in the weight room, so her sister invited her to try CrossFit. Barber was immediately hooked, and within months, she realized she could be competitive. "When I got into CrossFit, I had strong legs from being a runner, but I didn't have a lot of muscle definition on me," she says. "I'm long and limby and will always have these baby deer legs. Through eating properly and fueling myself in the way that was needed to compete, I saw myself with muscle and loved it."

But early in her career, she injured her back and discovered she had spina bifida, scoliosis, and a fractured L-5 vertebra. She was told she would never squat again, but she was determined to rebound better than ever. Barber knew she had a greater shot at protecting her vulnerable spine with strong muscles rather than weak ones. "I took that first year back from injury very, very slowly and learned how to listen to my body," she says. "I had to push a little in the beginning to figure out where that boundary was, where that red line was."

Barber didn't just squat again; she came back strong enough to put in multiple appearances at the CrossFit Games, standing on the podium a total of three times. "I didn't know if I would have the ability to compete at all again," she says. "It was icing on the cake of a recovery I just prayed for."

Doctors may have told Barber that lifting weights just wasn't for her, but what she learned through the experience is that weights are *definitely* for her. Limitations, on the other hand, are not.

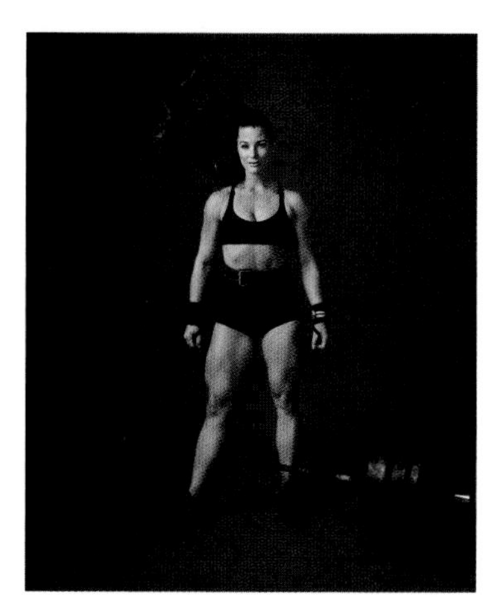

CAMILLE BROWN

WEIGHTLIFTER

BORN: 1992

HOMETOWN: Venice Beach, California

WHAT SHE'S KNOWN FOR: Brown has competed in Olympic weightlifting on a national level and is a certified personal trainer. She played softball at California Polytechnic State University.

As a kid, Camille Brown loved nothing more than playing softball. The only problem? She was small, slow, and not particularly powerful when it came to hitting or throwing. But she was undeterred, earning playing time by hustling on and off the field and cheering on her teammates. When she was in eighth grade, her dad enrolled her in a strength and conditioning program, in hopes that she'd at least get strong enough that if she slid into a bigger player, she wouldn't break anything. It was intimidating at first, especially because she was the only girl in the program, but she fell in love with the process. Over the next four years, she put on twenty-two pounds of muscle—not exactly a goal of her peers.

"I went to high school in Hollywood, where everybody's in tune with what's the latest fashion," she says. "I remember my friends saying, 'I just want my hip bones or collarbones or my rib cage to show.' I was sitting in class one day after hearing all these comments and feeling like maybe my rib cage should show. For the first time, I was really comparing myself to other females, thinking, 'Maybe I should tone it down on the training a little bit.' Then I snapped back and thought, 'No, I love that I can do pull-ups, hit the ball hard, sprint fast, and steal bases.'"

That mentality got her the dream: playing Division I softball. When Brown started lifting, she could only back squat a PVC pipe with five pounds on each side. She went to college with a back squat of 225 pounds. (It's now inching toward 300.)

More than just improving her physical power, strength training did wonders for her overall well-being. "Lifting weights has helped my mental state," she says. "Your anxiety goes down because you're so confident when you have X amount of weight on your back and you do a back squat and you've never done that before."

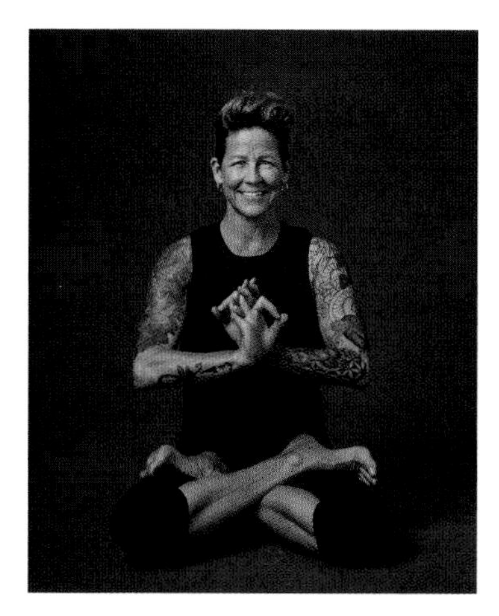

DANA TRIXIE FLYNN

YOGI

BORN: 1961

HOMETOWN: San Francisco, California

WHAT SHE'S KNOWN FOR: Flynn's New York City yoga studio, Laughing Lotus, turned twenty in 2019, and she also owns a generosity-based studio in New Orleans called the Church of Yoga.

From stockbroker to MTV reporter to clubby restaurant owner, Dana Trixie Flynn did not imagine early on that the yoga mat would call her the way it eventually did. She played tennis, basketball, volleyball, and soccer growing up, and she particularly loved to ride her bike, which felt like freedom. It's still her favorite mode of transportation.

"Right from the get-go, I was completely adventurous and outrageous, a wild child," she remembers. "I had all this energy and no direction, and later yoga gave me a chance to really focus all that energy and give it some good."

She took her first yoga class in New York in the late 1980s, but she wasn't yet ready for it. That would come a few years later, after she decided to get sober. She sold the Hell's Kitchen restaurant she owned, Trixies, which was filled with alcohol, her drug of choice. Then, she rediscovered yoga. This time, it stuck.

"When I got sober, I was looking around," she says. "Suddenly, at twenty-eight, I was going, 'What's it all about? Why am I here? How do I create change?' I knew a lot about a lot of things, but I didn't know anything about myself."

Flynn's contagious style of flow incorporates a love of dance, music, and movement; she describes it as "a wild moving prayer." "Yoga's not just stretching; it connects you with the divine," she says. "It's a body-mind-soul connection where the breath is the bridge between the body and the soul. For me, it really is a dance with God."

She ends every class with the words "Loving you, loving life, namaste."

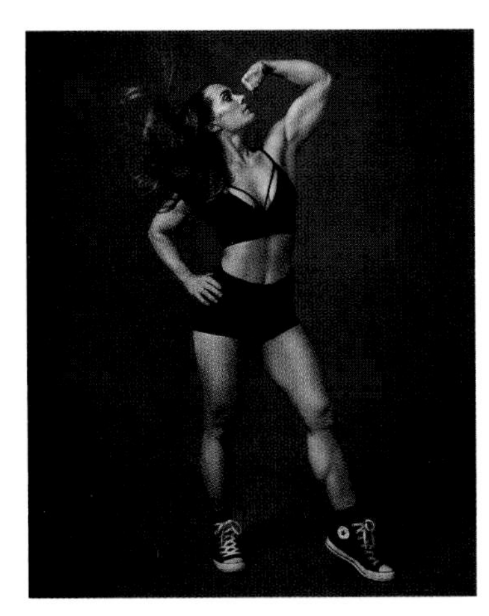

MEG GALLAGHER

POWERLIFTER

BORN: 1988

HOMETOWN: Akron, Ohio

WHAT SHE'S KNOWN FOR: Gallagher is a national-level powerlifter. At the 2018 USA Powerlifting Raw Nationals, she lifted a combined 402.5 kilograms (about 887 pounds) while competing in the 63-kilogram class. She also runs the popular YouTube channel MegSquats.

Growing up as a latchkey kid, Meg Gallagher had sports for a babysitter. After playing basketball and running cross-country in college, she fell into the pattern a lot of young professionals do: more happy hours, fewer workouts.

Fast-forward a few years, and Gallagher found her way to strength sports, going from CrossFit to bodybuilding to powerlifting, a sport in which she's competed at a national level. Initially, she was exercising to look better, but somewhere along the way, her outlook shifted. "For me, lifting weights did start as a physique goal," she says, "but once I started lifting more, I unlocked a gate to the strength world. It was easy to get hooked, and how I looked wasn't my priority anymore."

Through her YouTube channel and other social-media platforms, she works to disseminate sound information about building strength and facilitates honest discussions around body image. Now it's her mission to get a barbell into every woman's hands.

"I wasted so much time confused," she says. "I either went into the gym and avoided the weights or didn't go to the gym at all. I always felt like it was a chore or something to check off my list of things to do to get skinny. I was never going to the gym with the intention of being a badass, and now that's what I get to do every day."

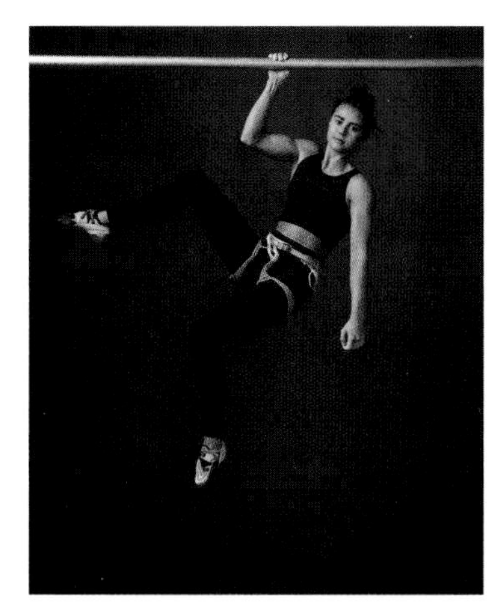

MARGO HAYES

CLIMBER

BORN: 1998

HOMETOWN: Boulder, Colorado

WHAT SHE'S KNOWN FOR: In 2017, Hayes became the first woman ever to climb a route graded 9a+ (5.15a): *La Rambla* in Spain. She's since climbed two other routes of equal difficulty, *Biographie* in France and *Papichulo* in Spain.

One of the top sport climbers in the world, Margo Hayes started her athletic career as a gymnast. She progressed quickly, catching the eye of USA Gymnastics and being invited to their talent development program. "I trained hard, set big goals—but didn't listen to my body," she says. Unfortunately, that resulted in multiple injuries that hampered her ability to work out.

While recovering from broken metatarsals at the age of ten, Hayes heard from a friend about climbing as a way to stay active without putting too much stress on her foot. She loved it. For a couple of years, she juggled gymnastics and climbing, before moving exclusively to her newfound sport at the age of twelve.

Since then, Hayes has made a big splash in the climbing world, pushing the limits of what can be achieved with an incredibly calm and methodical approach, unreal flexibility, and a fierce never-give-up attitude. "There is a lot of preparation before projecting a particular climb," she says. "Before climbing *La Rambla,* I read about the history of the route and watched other climbers on the line. It becomes part of you. You think about it, dream about it, and sometimes worry about it. To finally realize that goal after what feels like so many failed attempts is overwhelming. It is a combination of relief and elation. Those climbs, which require such dedication and commitment, I carry with me forever."

Despite her undeniable athletic ability, Hayes feels her true strength lies elsewhere. "The definition of *strength* to me surpasses physical prowess," she says. "I believe that staying true to my values, recognizing my weaknesses, and having compassion for others are my strengths."

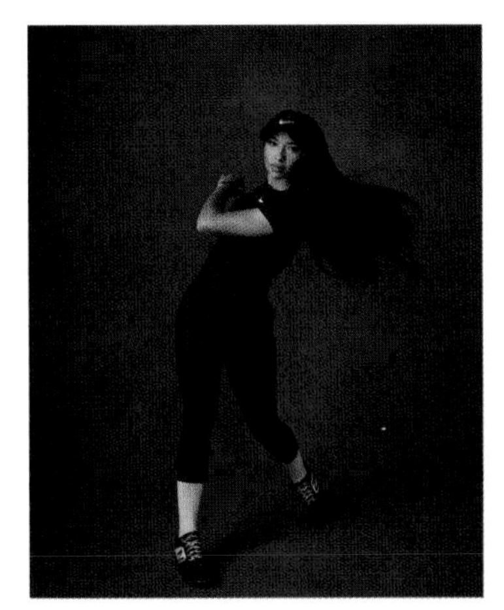

JAZMYN JACKSON

SOFTBALL PLAYER

BORN: 1996

HOMETOWN: San Jose, California

WHAT SHE'S KNOWN FOR: Jackson played softball at the University of California, Berkeley, where she racked up a slew of honors, including All-Pac-12 First Team. After graduating, she began coaching at Howard University and has been a member of the U.S. national team since 2016.

When Jazmyn Jackson's parents saw that she had a talent for softball, they made sure she was never the best person on the team. That required Jackson to stretch her abilities, playing with girls who were older and had more experience, but it meant she never rested on her laurels. She was always striving for more.

"I love that softball is absolutely one of the hardest games to play," she says. "Hitting the ball three times out of ten is a good statistic, which kind of blows my mind because that's not how I run my life. You have to learn to deal with failure—you're forced to have a short memory because you fail so much."

To train in quickness and explosiveness, Jackson lifts weights three to four times a week, focusing on hang cleans, bench presses, and accessory work. She also does conditioning drills, such as running sprints. "You can never master this game—that's why you see baseball players only get better as the years go by," she says. "I learn something every single day, and that's really cool for me."

Softball is an enduring passion for Jackson, but it's also been a lifesaver. After she found herself in an abusive relationship, she tried to shrink away, becoming quieter and smaller and avoiding attention and compliments.

When she was traveling with the national softball team, though, she was free to be herself, and she realized how joyful that made her. Jackson decided enough was enough. "You build strength by going through hard times," she says. "Being able to be a failure on the field and still be happy and able to lift myself up out of a dark situation is being strong."

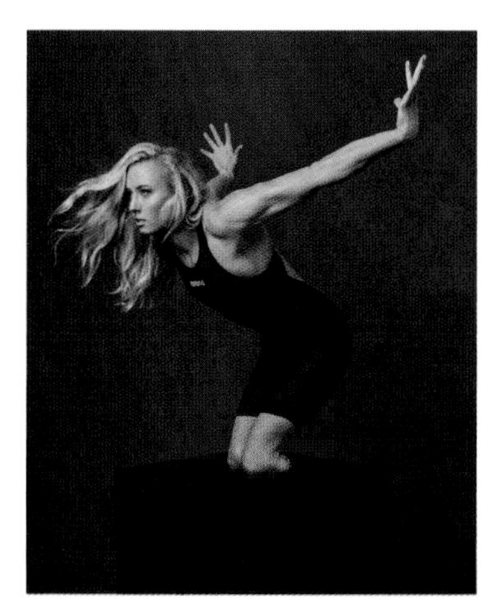

JESSICA LONG

PARALYMPIC SWIMMER

BORN: 1992

HOMETOWN: Baltimore, Maryland

WHAT SHE'S KNOWN FOR: Over the course of four Paralympics, Long has won twenty-three medals, thirteen of them gold. She has set multiple world records and was the first (and so far only) Paralympian to win the AAU Sullivan Award, which has been given to the best amateur athlete in the United States every year since 1930.

When Jessica Long was a young girl, she was mesmerized by the movie *The Little Mermaid*. "Here was this mermaid who wanted legs, and I remember being like, 'Oh my gosh, I can relate,' " she says. "I always wanted legs but knew I was never going to have them."

Born in Siberia with a rare birth defect known as fibular hemimelia, Long had her lower legs amputated at eighteen months old. She was placed in an orphanage by her teenage mother and adopted by an American couple.

Although the combination of a disability, adoption, and even a birthday on

Leap Day made Long feel different growing up, she found success and solace in sports. "I was always very competitive, and honestly, I think that drive came from not having my lower legs," she says. "Part of me always felt in this crazy way that I just had to prove myself."

In 2004, she went to the Paralympic Games in Athens at the age of twelve, the youngest competitor there. No one expected her to make the team, given that she'd only been swimming competitively for two years at that point. "I honestly think what set me apart was that I just had a whole different way of understanding the water," she says. "One of the most beautiful things about the sport of swimming is that you can be this huge, strong man with lots of muscle, but if you don't understand the water, you're not going to move in the water. Even when I was young, I worked really hard on technique, and that's what gave me that little edge."

One should never underestimate a mermaid.

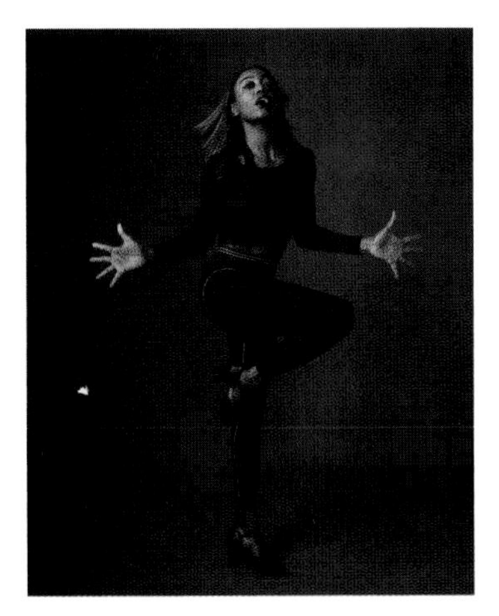

PATINA MILLER

ACTOR AND DANCER

BORN: 1984

HOMETOWN: Pageland, South Carolina

WHAT SHE'S KNOWN FOR: Miller is a 2013 Tony Award winner for Best Actress in a Musical, for the very physical (and traditionally male) role of the Leading Player in *Pippin*.

Nine years ago, Patina Miller wasn't so sure about lifting heavy weights. But after working with a trainer, she quickly changed her mind, as she realized all the benefits of getting strong—and how lifting more than twenty pounds didn't have to mean changing her body in a way she didn't want. "At first I thought, 'I can't lift weights, because I'm going to bulk and look like a man,' " she says. "Weights equaled 'masculine,' weights equaled 'women can't do that.' "

Her new mentality came in quite handy for her character in *Pippin*. For that, she wanted to both *look* strong and *be* strong, to walk the line between male and female energy, to fly through the air on the trapeze with confidence. And while Broadway might not technically be a sport, it certainly feels like one. "It's like running a marathon," Miller says. "Your mind and your body and your voice have to be able to withstand the strenuous task of performing eight times a week. People pay money to come and see you, so you do whatever you can do to meet the demands of that. You have to think like an athlete."

For someone who's always found endorphins through exercise and expression through movement, working out also helped Miller keep a piece of herself after her daughter was born in 2017.

"Postpartum depression is a big thing after having a baby," she says. "The saving grace for me for the first year was moving my body and being in the gym. It definitely was my therapy. It was not about me being selfish, it was not about me being full of myself, it really was for my sanity. That hour a day I could get away from feeling dark, feeling down—that was my high."

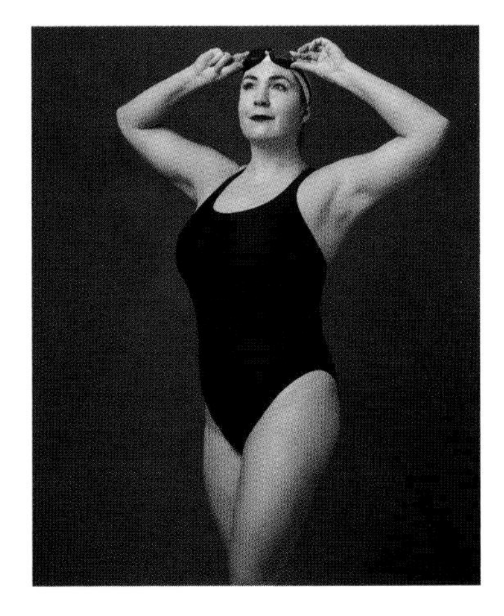

JAIMIE MONAHAN

ENDURANCE AND ICE SWIMMER

BORN: 1979

HOMETOWN: Ossining, New York

WHAT SHE'S KNOWN FOR: A seven-time U.S. national champion in winter swimming, Monahan is a member of both the International Marathon Swimming Hall of Fame and the International Ice Swimming Hall of Fame, and she has twice been named Woman of the Year by the World Open Water Swimming Association. In 2018, she swam six marathons on six continents in sixteen days, a Guinness World Record, and she is the first person to complete the Ice Sevens Challenge, one mile on each continent in sub-41-degree water.

Jaimie Monahan's swimming background is fairly traditional. She got started in the pool as a wee one, then went on to swim in college before tapering off in adulthood. After working on Wall Street for many years, she took up running marathons and then competing in triathlons, eventually building up to the Ironman distance (2.4-mile swim, 112-mile bike ride, 26.2-mile run). That's when the story takes a less conventional turn. From there, she trained to swim the English Channel in 2009, which opened the door to challenges such as ice swimming and marathons (defined as anything more than 10k in the water).

Monahan describes being submerged in the water as a comfortable feeling, but it does occasionally come with some unwelcome surprises. When she was swimming in Alexandria, Egypt, in 2018, she started to see beautiful jellyfish floating by. "The first one hit, and it felt like I was being electrocuted," she says. "Later I got another one—it kind of wrapped around me. I felt like my hand was slammed in a car door; it actually felt like my flesh was ripped away. I had to look at my arm to make sure there wasn't a chunk out of me."

Fortunately, those kinds of moments are the exception to the rule. The longer she's out there, the better—Monahan particularly enjoys swims that last more than twenty-four hours. "Facing these physical challenges is great," she says, "because I can say, 'Hey, I've already swum in ice water this week. Anything that work comes to me with or situations I have to solve, I feel pretty confident I can take whatever's coming to me.' "

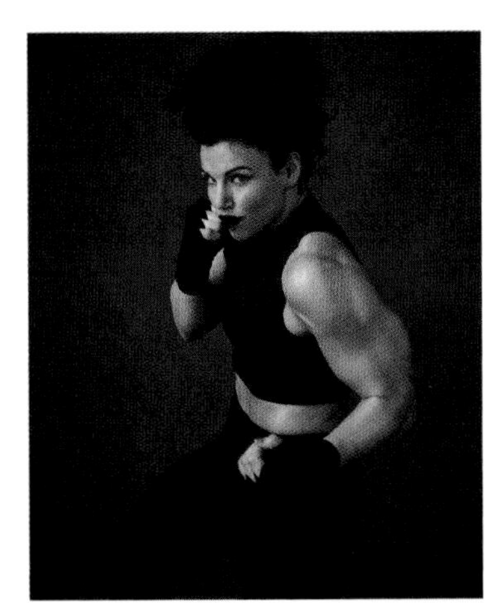

ALICIA NAPOLEON-ESPINOSA

BOXER

BORN: 1986

HOMETOWN: Manorville, New York

WHAT SHE'S KNOWN FOR: Napoleon-Espinosa is a World Boxing Association super middleweight women's world champion and cofounder of Overthrow Boxing Club. In 2018, she was named Breakout Fighter of the Year. Her professional record is 12-1, with seven knockouts.

Alicia Napoleon-Espinosa didn't always have the easiest time growing up. "In school, I had big hips, big lips, and thick, long, black, curly hair," she says. "I definitely developed a lot sooner than most of the girls, and people called me Thunder Thighs. I wasn't the girl that the boy would have the crush on. I just wasn't like the rest of them. I always loved my legs and I always loved my shape, but there were definitely moments I would get really upset about it and I would feel embarrassed."

The Empress, as she's now known, says she came out of the womb in love with boxing, but it wasn't until she was eighteen that she found a gym where she could train. Until that point, the self-described girly tomboy danced, did karate, played basketball and volleyball, wrestled, and was captain of the cheer team. Her early dream was to become a professional baseball player, but she was told that would never happen since she was a girl.

Alongside fighting in the ring, she considers it equally important to fight against those norms that say what a woman can and can't be. "Embrace who you are," Napoleon-Espinosa says. "Make the best you—all shapes and sizes, all ethnicities, all colors. God has a plan and he built us all beautiful."

Through all the criticism, she's never let the fact that she's a woman stop her from pursuing what's often considered a masculine sport. "I'm an aggressive and passionate person," she says. "I do have my moments where I'm calm and tranquil, but I can be a force, and this has helped me find stability. It's been very therapeutic. I'm probably going to box until the day I die."

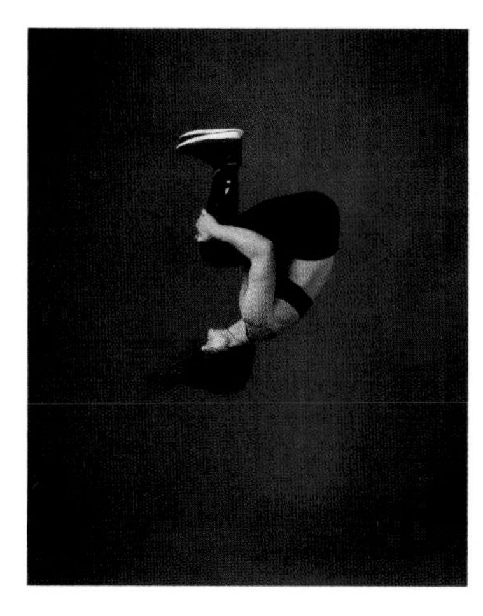

SYDNEY OLSON

FREERUNNER

BORN: 1993

HOMETOWN: Port Orchard, Washington

WHAT SHE'S KNOWN FOR: Olson is a professional freerunner sponsored by Tempest and Yokohama, and she works as a stuntwoman for television shows.

As a teenager, Sydney Olson was introduced to the world of parkour and freerunning, sports that involve negotiating one's surroundings to run, jump, climb, and flip as efficiently (parkour) or stylishly (freerunning) as possible. Seven years of competitive gymnastics gave her some advantages, but she was actually attracted to the fact that it wasn't easy to conquer all the moves. Needing to break down the technique made it more rewarding when she did master a new skill.

"I was pretty horrible at some of the basics, but it just made me want to get better," she says. "The idea that there was always something I could improve on with it appealed to me. It became my entire life eventually."

But first, there were some mental hurdles to clear in a sport that's dominated by men. "When I started parkour, there weren't a lot of girls at all, really almost none," Olson says. "I had it in my head for a while that girls just weren't good at it. I thought, 'I'm not gonna be as good as the guys.' I just had a switch in my head, and I said, 'I can keep working hard and try the same things they're doing and do whatever I want.' Over time, I learned not to limit myself in that way."

To stay at the top of the freerunning game, Olson incorporates weightlifting, powerlifting, and Olympic lifting into her routine, along with conditioning classes, judo, and kickboxing. Not only has training to move functionally helped her excel in her career, but it's also put to rest body insecurities she had in her youth.

"I was really self-conscious back then, and I did not like wearing shorts," she remembers. "If you're struggling with body image, it can go away. Your self-worth shouldn't be defined by the way you look."

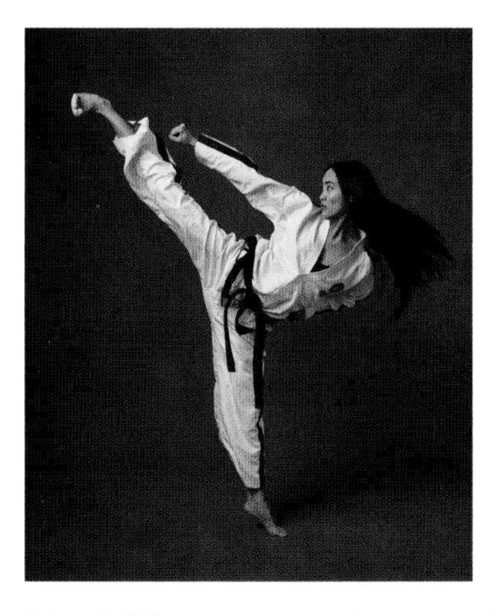

STEPHANIE PHAM

MARTIAL ARTIST

BORN: 1992

HOMETOWN: Philadelphia, Pennsylvania

WHAT SHE'S KNOWN FOR: Pham is a fourth-degree black belt who competed in two World Taekwondo Championships and two World Cup Taekwondo Championships.

Stephanie Pham's father had always wanted his children to practice martial arts. When Pham was seven, she got that opportunity. But her introduction to taekwondo was not an immediate hit. She cried on her first day at what she thought looked like a very scary activity.

Yet it took just a couple of weeks until she was completely hooked. "I was very driven to want to be the best," she says. "It's not hard to get lost in something if you're passionate."

The petite Pham is proof that appearances can be deceiving. She had a lot of naysayers who didn't believe how good she was. Instead of getting defensive, she let her skills do the talking. "Growing up, a lot of people were like, 'You can't fight; you're so small,'" she says. "I was like, 'OK, I don't have anything to prove to you because I do fight, and it hurts. I fight men, and you can talk to those guys.'"

For Pham, taekwondo practice went well beyond the mat, permeating all areas of her life. "If you're a martial artist and you meet another martial artist, there's that level of respect that's already kind of there. It doesn't matter how old you are or what race you are, you have a way to connect and something to talk about even if it's a different style," she says. "Courtesy, integrity, perseverance, self-control, indomitable spirit—all those core values we learn in martial arts, we're actually expected to practice. Overall, it makes you a better person. I am who I am today because of it."

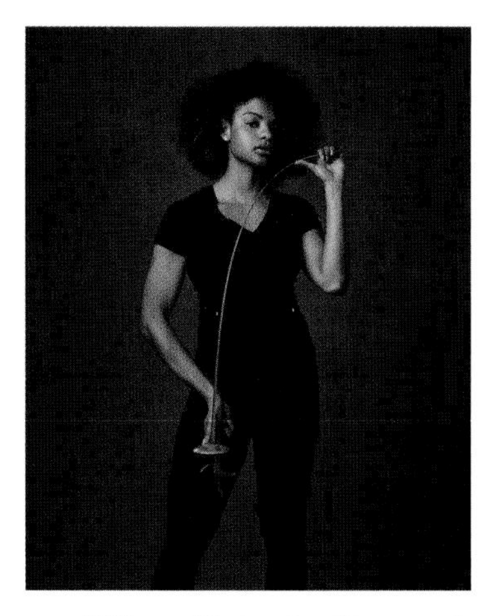

NZINGHA PRESCOD

FENCER

BORN: 1992

HOMETOWN: Brooklyn, New York

WHAT SHE'S KNOWN FOR: Prescod competed in both the 2012 London and 2016 Rio Olympics in foil fencing, and she was the first African American woman ever to win an individual medal at the Senior World Fencing Championships.

When Nzingha Prescod was nine, her mom heard about a program called the Peter Westbrook Foundation that was producing black Olympians in fencing. Prescod had always been athletic, so she gave it a go, but it wasn't love at first lunge. The stance was awkward and uncomfortable to learn, and the coaches were insistent that there was only one way the legs should be, one way the arms should be, one way to hold a weapon. That wasn't something Prescod was used to in the other sports she'd tried, but she soon came to love fencing and dedicated herself to becoming as good at it as possible.

After two Olympic Games appearances and a nagging injury, she left the sport, but her life felt empty without it. "I started working this internship in consulting," she says. "I was traveling, and I would go to my hotel after work and be back at seven, then I'd be like, 'What do I do now?' I didn't have anything I was pursuing; it was just go to work and then watch *The Bachelor*—which is cool, I like to watch *The Bachelor*, but doing that and then doing that again, I was like, 'I can't do it,' so I started fencing again with goals of going beyond what I had already achieved."

Medals are still great, but now that she's older, Prescod's perspective has shifted. She understands that fencing has brought much more to her life than just accolades, and she knows it still has more to offer. "In my adult career, my motivation comes from personal development," she says. "I don't want to be a timid person; I want to be vocal and expressive, and I want to have a voice. Now I'm fencing with the goal of being courageous."

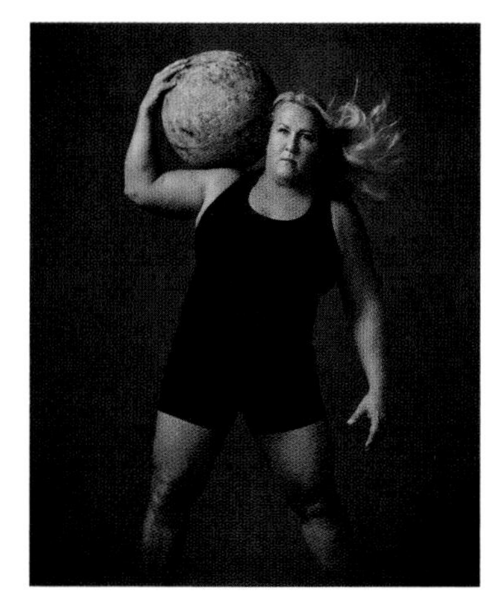

KRISTIN RHODES

STRONGWOMAN

BORN: 1975

HOMETOWN: San Diego, California

WHAT SHE'S KNOWN FOR: Rhodes is the 2012 World's Strongest Woman and eight-time America's Strongest Woman. In 2019, she broke the world record for the circus dumbbell press, at 175 pounds.

There were early signs that Kristin Rhodes possessed great strength—as a baby, she liked to pick up heavy stuff and carry it around for fun, and she was a thrower in college—but it wasn't until she was thirty that she found her way to strongwoman competitions.

Although she started training for her sport later in life than many other athletes, she's only getting better with time. "What's kind of mind-blowing to me at this point is I just keep getting stronger—I'm kind of defying science," she says. "With every year, I continue to get stronger, so I don't even know where my max is going to be."

To stay dominant in a demanding sport—565-pound deadlifts do have a way of taxing the body—Rhodes is conscientious about taking care of herself. "I'm very good at self-regulating, and if I feel like my body needs a break, I'll take a break," she says. "There have been times where after a competition, I'll take two, three, four months off, and I won't lift at all, because I just kind of need that mental and physical break."

Rhodes has always fit her training around the demands of raising three kids. She remembers times where she'd run back and forth from the kitchen to the garage gym, preparing dinner and getting in a few sets simultaneously. The juggling act was worth it—not only has she been incredibly successful in competitions, but she's also shown her children that with hard work, anything is possible.

"It's pretty surreal to say that I'm literally one of the strongest women in the world," she says. "It's humbling. To think this small girl from San Diego has accomplished this big feat of strength is pretty amazing."

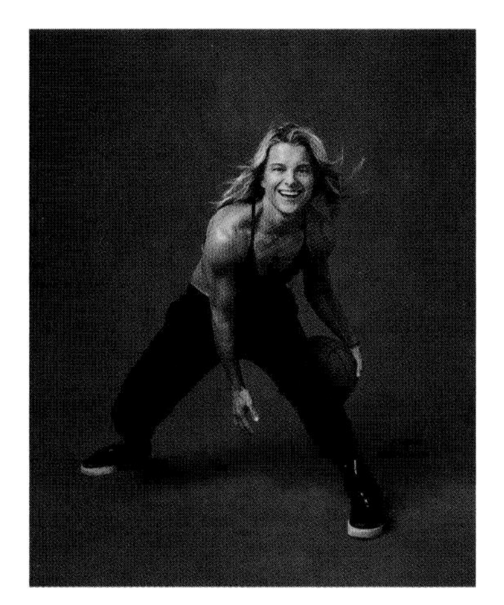

HOLLY RILINGER

BASKETBALL PLAYER AND TRAINER

BORN: 1974

HOMETOWNS: Lincoln, Nebraska and Waynesboro, Virginia

WHAT SHE'S KNOWN FOR: Rilinger played pro basketball before becoming a Nike Master Trainer. She appeared on the Bravo show *Work Out New York* and is the author of the fitness book *Lifted*.

From a young age, Holly Rilinger gravitated toward basketball. In seventh grade, when her family moved and she went from a private Catholic school to a public school, it became her saving grace. In the halls, she felt judged, but on the court, she was somebody. Rilinger went on to lead her high school team to the state championship in her senior year and was recruited by hundreds of colleges. After a successful collegiate career, she played professionally overseas and was picked up as a free agent by the WNBA's Phoenix Mercury—quite a feat for someone just five-foot-four—before injury dashed her dreams.

"I certainly had plenty of people tell me that maybe I should consider another sport; just because I was so athletic, I could've been great at a lot of things where my height didn't put me at a disadvantage," Rilinger says. "But if I'd chosen another sport, I would've never wanted to practice as much as the sport I was insanely passionate about."

Post-basketball, Rilinger was lost. After some trial and error, she found her way into personal training. Today she teaches a variety of classes, including Lifted, her own blend of high-intensity intervals and meditation. "A turning point for me was when I found spin," she says. "I felt like a point guard again, getting up in the front of the room with fifty people in front of me, leading them in the same way I might've led my team. My dad says my gift is saying the right things at the right time. The moment comes, and I'm out of breath, and the words come because I've lived it—it's genuine and it's real."

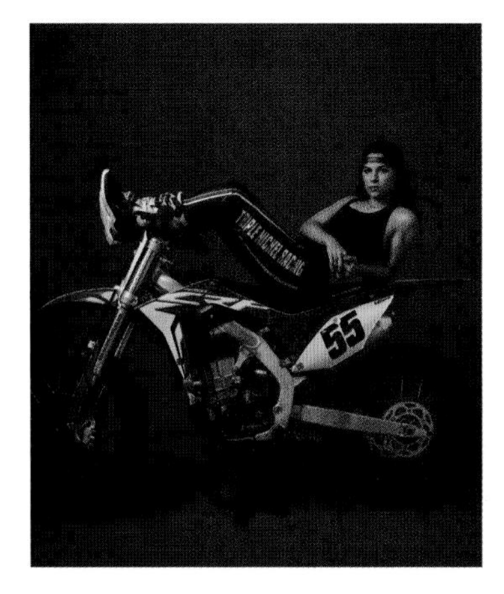

SANDRIANA SHIPMAN

FLAT-TRACK MOTORCYCLE RACER

BORN: 1995

HOMETOWN: Maybrook, New York

WHAT SHE'S KNOWN FOR: Shipman is one of just two women who compete in flat-track racing on a professional level.

Sandriana Shipman has twelve first cousins, mostly boys, and they all grew up riding anything and everything they could find. But no one—including parents, aunts, and uncles—ever raced seriously. After Shipman's dad took her to a flat-track motorcycle race when she was seven, the competitive fire was lit, and every weekend from there on out, they were off at another race.

Flat track is fast and furious, and with that comes plenty of risk. "We're going one hundred miles per hour inches from each other, slinging the bike completely sideways for twenty-five laps," she says. "It's like NASCAR except we don't have cages—there's nothing between the ground and us. It's speed, it's intensity, it's on the edge of your seat, it makes your heart skip. We just go."

The inherent danger is not lost on Shipman, who has broken her back three times, along with an ankle, a wrist, and fingers, to name just a few of her bones that have caught an unlucky break. She's torn a rotator cuff, bruised a lung, and lacerated her liver. A large scar runs down her femur.

Still, she's undeterred. "I keep putting myself out there," she says. "Other people, when they get hurt, they tend to shy away and slow down and take it easy and wait for their mentality to come back, but I've never really had that issue."

There are obstacles beyond the physical. The sport is expensive, and Shipman's had to DIY her career more than most. After making her professional debut in American Flat Track in 2017, she rolled up to the races with a car and a lawn mower trailer carrying her bike—not the ideal setup. Against the odds, she's proven with quick times that she belongs on the racing oval, battered bones and all. Her motivation? Pure love of the sport.

"I'm not big on being in the media and being a name," Shipman says. "I wanted to go pro so I could race on that level with those people on the cooler tracks." If she can inspire a few young girls along the way, all the better.

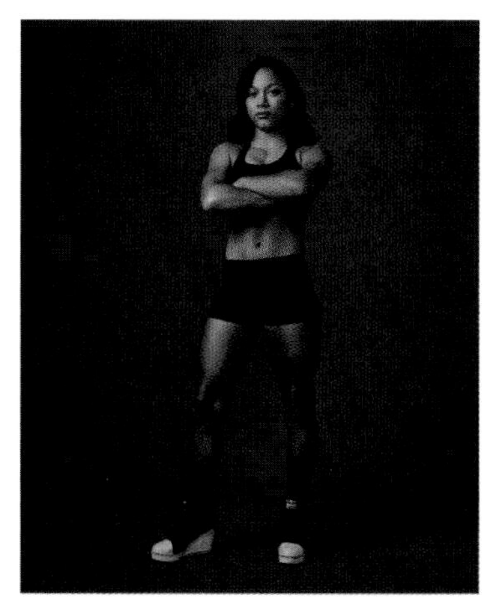

DAMIYAH SMITH

ALL-AROUND ATHLETE

BORN: 2006

HOMETOWN: Commerce, Oklahoma

WHAT SHE'S KNOWN FOR: Smith is an Oklahoma state champion in powerlifting and excels at several sports. She can squat more than 225 pounds, bench more than 145 pounds, and deadlift more than 260 pounds.

After noticing that their daughter was oddly strong for a baby, Damiyah Smith's parents thought she was destined for gymnastics. She didn't take to that sport, but once she picked up a barbell at age eight, it became clear that powerlifting was an activity in which she could truly shine.

Among the weight racks, she's found a sense of belonging. "I like that going to the gym makes me feel good about myself," she says. "I used to have a little insecurity because I was bullied."

Known as the Powerhouse Princess, the middle schooler is racking up the records in powerlifting and weightlifting—she's up to thirty-six and has a goal of one hundred of them before she graduates from high school. Determined to reach that mark, Smith wakes up around five each morning all on her own in order to get to the gym before school. "I like to inspire people," she says. "It makes me feel really good that people look up to me."

After classes are done for the day, she's back to working out. Boxing, basketball, wrestling, and track are just a few of her other pursuits. As if all that weren't enough, Smith also started a line of sports nutrition supplements for kids. One day, she hopes to compete in the Olympics.

"Never give up, because once you start something, you've gotta keep going," she says. "If you give up the first time because it's hard, you're never going to accomplish anything."

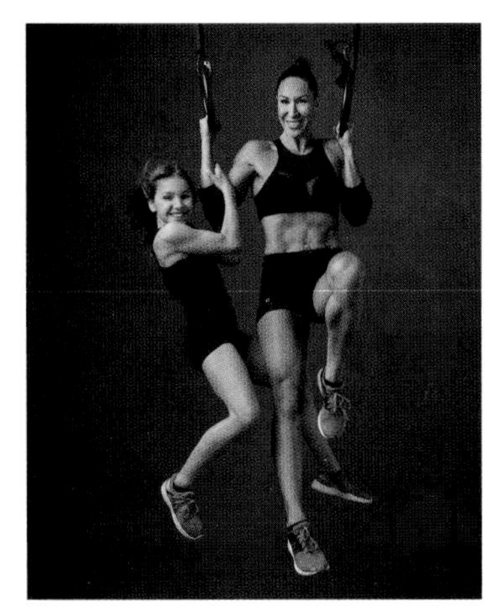

MAGGI THORNE

***AMERICAN NINJA WARRIOR* COMPETITOR**

BORN: 1981

HOMETOWN: San Diego, California

WHAT SHE'S KNOWN FOR: Thorne has competed on five seasons of TV's *American Ninja Warrior*. She also appeared on *Spartan: Ultimate Team Challenge* and was a collegiate track star.

When Maggi Thorne was fourteen, a PE teacher noticed that she looked as if she might be fast. The track coaches invited her to try out for the team, which changed the trajectory of her life. Growing up,

Thorne's family was low-income; they shared a home with another family. Both her brothers were dropouts, and even though she struggled with academics, she was determined to forge a different path. "I always knew I had the fire to try things and to not sell myself short," she says. "I had to be willing to climb mountains when I had no idea what was ahead."

Thorne went to junior college, got an associate's degree, and became a California state champion in hurdles before being heavily recruited by universities. All through college, tough situations kept following her, from an abusive relationship to sexual assault to divorce to losing her track scholarship at the University of Nebraska due to poor performance. She persevered and continued to compete despite losing the scholarship, earning her way to the national championships in both indoor and outdoor track as a senior. Then she got a dream job designing athletic facilities and managing construction projects, but when her best friend committed suicide, she felt called to build people instead of buildings. When she thought of the skills and gifts she had and how to best put those to use, *American Ninja Warrior* seemed like the perfect platform to reach others—and it also turned out to be a great source of support.

"Once you step into the *Ninja* community, you fall in love with it," she says. "It's like family. A lot of us have a large group chat, and we let other people know about opportunities to compete at events or work with companies. We also offer encouragement. This isn't an everyone-out-for-themselves sport."

The *ANW* competitor, obstacle-course racer, and mother of three now works to spread a message of empowerment and encouragement to as many people as she can. "There's that physical strength that everybody can see," Thorne says, "but when you can find your inner strength and own it and celebrate it, that is when you're going to come alive."

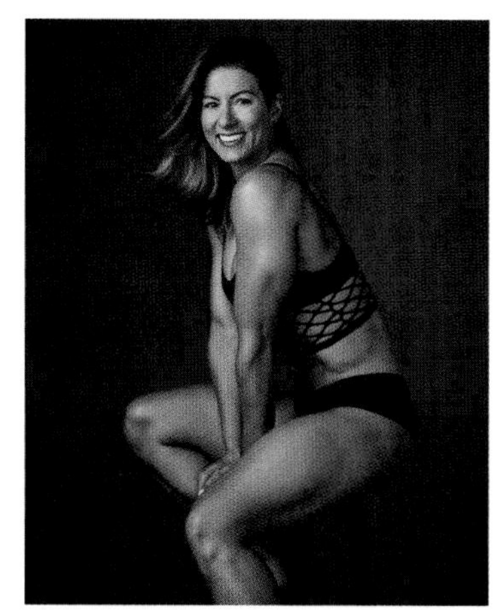

JEN WIDERSTROM

FITNESS TRAINER

BORN: 1982

HOMETOWN: Downers Grove, Illinois

WHAT SHE'S KNOWN FOR: Widerstrom appeared on TV's *American Gladiators* and *The Biggest Loser.* She's the best-selling author of *Diet Right for Your Personality Type* and the fitness director for *Shape* magazine.

Before she became an undefeated coach on *The Biggest Loser,* before she intimidated contenders as Phoenix on *American Gladiators,* before she graced the cover of countless fitness magazines, Jen Widerstrom was a kid from the Chicago suburbs who just liked to move.

She didn't always have the words to express herself, but when she was engaged in movement and physical exertion—she never saw it as exercise—she built confidence and her own voice.

Her big break was on *American Gladiators.* After it was canceled, she felt adrift and started to work as a trainer as a way to pay her bills. "What was fascinating to me was so much more than people's results," she says. "I could see movement affecting the way they felt about themselves: making better eye contact, walking a little taller, choosing a brighter shirt to train in. That's where I started to really fall in love with using this vehicle of fitness, of movement, to have deeper conversations, facilitate deeper transformations, and foster a deeper connection with people to help them find themselves again, or perhaps for the first time."

As sad as she felt about the ending of *American Gladiators,* Widerstrom realized it was a gift. On the show, she dressed up and played a character. Now she had the opportunity to show the world who she really was.

She subsequently found her voice in the fitness industry as a positive presence who meets people where they are. Instead of instilling fear in her clients, she empowers them to take pride in their health journey. “There’s nothing stronger than standing in who you are and doing it on purpose,” she says. “The whole world will change around you.”

ABOUT THE AUTHOR

Haley Shapley is a journalist whose writing has appeared in *The Saturday Evening Post, Rachael Ray Every Day, SELF, American Way,* Shape.com, and *The Telegraph.* An Olympics superfan and exercise enthusiast, Shapley has cycled 206 miles from Seattle to Portland, summited the highest glaciated peak in the continental United States, competed in a bodybuilding show, and run a marathon. She lives in Seattle.

ACKNOWLEDGMENTS

A book like this would not be possible without, pardon the pun, an extremely strong team. First on that list has to be my agent, Kate Johnson, who believed in this idea from day one and was always willing to weigh in on my many quandaries. I'm certain I would've been even less graceful throughout this process without her guidance.

A big thank-you to my editor, Karyn Marcus, for steering the ship. Her vision and thoughtful edits brought out the best in the material, and I consider myself incredibly lucky that we've had the opportunity to work together.

I'm indebted to everyone who generously shared their stories and expertise with me through interviews: Kim Beckwith, Randy Boelsems, Elaine Craig, Katrin Davidsdottir, Janet M. Davis, Edie Edmundson, Molly Galbraith, Louise Hazel, Liefia Ingalls, Nikki Lee, Linda Lin, Karyn Marshall, Nicole Mericle, Greg Nuckols, Jasmin Paris, Barclay Stockett, Meg Stone, Kathrine Switzer, Tia-Clair Toomey, Lei Wang, and Steve Wennerstrom. Whether it was for fifteen minutes or three hours, every conversation I had in some way shaped the book.

That group of interviewees also includes the twenty-three women whose portraits appear throughout these pages, who carved time out of their busy schedules to attend the photo shoots and show their particular brands of strength. Meeting them all was one of the highlights of the process—and a huge dose of inspiration.

The photo shoots buzzed with a palpable energy, and that's thanks to my partner in crime, Sophy Holland. I'm grateful she agreed to be part of this project—

she understood the message from the very beginning and assembled incredible crews to create gorgeous photos that help bring the words to life. It was so fun to work with Kendall Gough, whose fangirl enthusiasm matched my own.

Thank you to the Seattle Public Library for hosting me in the Writers' Room. The H. J. Lutcher Stark Center for Physical Culture and Sports was a helpful spot for research, and I greatly appreciate all of librarian Cindy Slater's assistance in navigating the materials. Thanks also to Alyssa Wynans for stepping in to help verify facts. Closer to home, the members at Riot Athletics were always willing to take yet another survey, and their enthusiasm surrounding the book was a welcome source of energy for me.

I'm grateful to Rebecca Strobel, Marla Dunn, Ashley Wilson, and Molly Gregory for providing feedback on the manuscript at various stages. Thank you to Emily Boynton for jumping in headfirst on a tight timeline to assist with research and fact-checking.

I'd be remiss if I didn't give credit to Kai, who's been with me every step along the way, even though his interest in books ends at knocking them off countertops. Special thanks to Tobias the Owl, Jim Stein, and Henry Photangtham, who helped make it possible for me to travel when needed.

And finally, I wouldn't be where I am without my family's support. My mom carted me around to endless sports practices and competitions when I was growing up, and even when she doesn't understand the athletic challenges I set for myself, she always shows up to watch me cross the finish line anyway. When I first mentioned the book idea to her and my sister, Chelsea, they immediately told me I had to pursue it. Had they not, it may have ended there. I've truly valued my sister's wisdom (despite the fact that, yes, I am the older, wiser one) and belief that I'm capable of anything. Deepest thanks to my entire family for being the earliest supporters of *Strong Like Her*—and of me.

HISTORICAL PHOTO CREDITS

P. 17 Villa Romana del Casale mosaic: Konstantin Kalishko © 123RF.com

P. 26 Ada Anderson: *Frank Leslie's Illustrated Newspaper*, Brooklyn Collection, Brooklyn Public Library

P. 44 Annette Kellermann: Library of Congress, Prints & Photographs Division, LC-DIG-ggbain-03569

P. 55 Sandwina: Library of Congress, Prints & Photographs Division, LC-DIG-ggbain-06840

P. 62 Frances Willard: Courtesy of the WCTU Archives, Evanston, Illinois

P. 70 Pudgy Stockton: Pudgy & Les Stockton Collection/Stark Center/University of Texas

P. 90 Babe Didrikson: AP/Shutterstock

P. 102 Kathrine Switzer: *Boston Herald*

P. 122 Jan Todd: Terry & Jan Todd Collection/Stark Center/University of Texas

P. 127 Karyn Marshall: Bruce Klemens Photo

P. 140 Elaine Craig: Steve Wennerstrom

P. 148 Simone Biles: Ulrik Pedersen/CSM/Shutterstock

P. 160 Lei Wang: Courtesy of Lei Wang

P. 173 Alex Morgan and Megan Rapinoe: TOLGA BOZOGLU/EPA-EFE/Shutterstock

PORTRAIT CREDITS

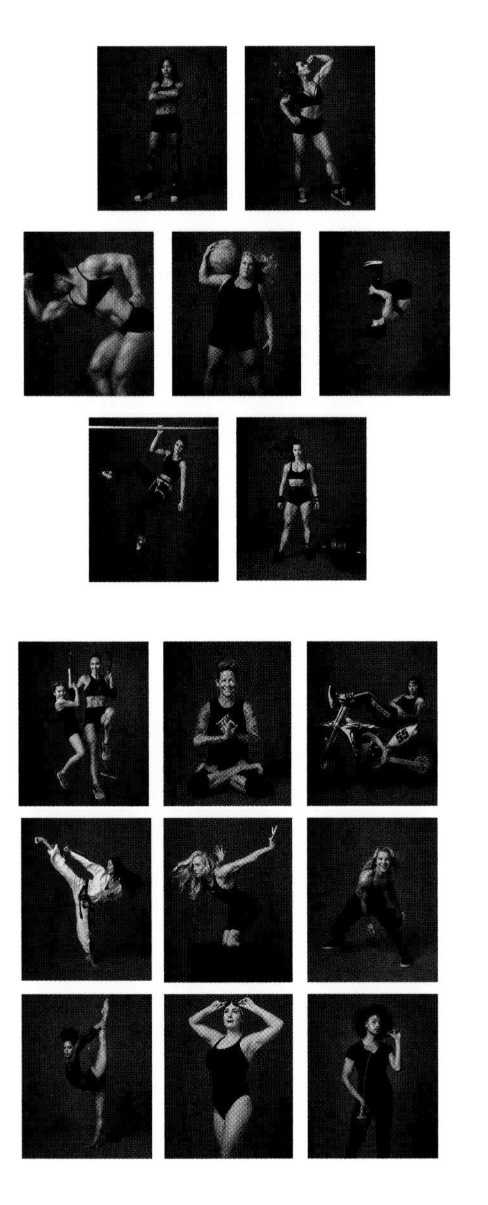

LIGHTING AND GRIP: Robb Epifano, Sam Velazquez

PRODUCTION COORDINATOR: Kendall Gough

HAIR: Sheridan Ward

MAKEUP: Caitlin Krenz

STUDIO: Smashbox Studios

BACKDROP: Schmidli Backdrops

LIGHTING AND GRIP: Henry Lopez, Richard Rose

PRODUCTION COORDINATOR: Kendall Gough

HAIR: Erin Tierney

MAKEUP: Shirley Pinkson

STUDIO: Pier59 Studios

BACKDROP: Schmidli Backdrops

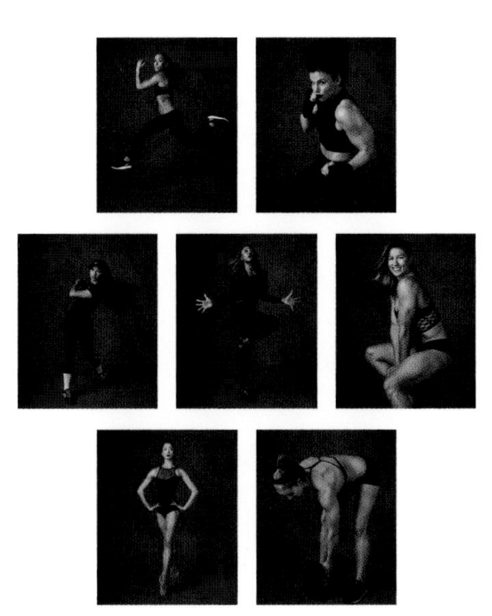

LIGHTING AND GRIP: Javier Villegas, Matt Stevens

PRODUCTION COORDINATOR: Kendall Gough

HAIR: Deycke Heidorn

MAKEUP: Colleen Runne

STUDIO: Pier59 Studios

BACKDROP: Schmidli Backdrops

NOTES

INTRODUCTION

2 *"At first sight":* Roger Ebert, review of *Pumping Iron II: The Women,* directed by George Butler, RogerEbert.com, May 31, 1985, https://www.rogerebert.com/reviews/pumping-iron-ii-the-women-1985.

3 *"I thought lifting was so cool":* Kristin Rhodes, interview with author, February 18, 2019.

CHAPTER 1

9 *Mount Typaeum:* John Mouratidis, "Heracles at Olympia and the Exclusion of Women from the Ancient Olympic Games," *Journal of Sport History* 11, no. 3 (Winter 1984): 50–53, www.jstor.org/stable/43609113.

10 *Heraean Games:* Shirsho Dasgupta, "Cynisca and the Heraean Games: The Female Athletes of Ancient Greece," *Wire,* August 21, 2016, https://thewire.in/history/cynisca-and-the-heraean-games-the-female-athletes-of-ancient-greece.

10 *Callipateira:* Thomas F. Scanlon, "Games for Girls," *Archaeology* 49, no. 4 (July/August 1996): 32–33, www.jstor.org/stable/41771026.

10 *Cynisca:* Anthony Everitt, *The Rise of Athens: The Story of the World's Greatest Civilization* (New York: Random House, 2016): 20–21.

11 *"I declare myself the only woman":* Everitt, *The Rise of Athens,* 20.

11 *The point was that wealth:* Donald G. Kyle, " 'The Only Woman in All Greece': Kyniska, Agesilaus, Alcibiades and Olympia," *Journal of Sport History* 30, no. 2 (Summer 2003): 183–203, www.jstor.org/stable/43610326.

11 *Philosopher Xenophon said this:* Sharon L. James and Sheila Dillon, eds., *A Companion to Women in the Ancient World* (Chichester: John Wiley & Sons, 2015): 16.

11 *Confirmed by biographer Plutarch:* Plutarch, *The Parallel Lives,* trans. Bernadotte Perrin (Loeb Classical Library): 247, http://penelope.uchicago.edu/Thayer/E/Roman/Texts/Plutarch/Lives/Lycurgus*.html.

12 *"No Spartan girl":* Allen Guttmann, *Women's Sports: A History* (New York: Columbia University Press, 1991): 27.

12 *"The most ridiculous thing of all":* Plato, *Plato's Republic,* trans. Benjamin Jowett (North Charleston, SC: CreateSpace): 242.

13 *Plato . . . dismissed the concern:* Betty Spears, "A Perspective of the History of Women's Sport in Ancient Greece," *Journal of Sport History* 11, no. 2 (Summer 1984): 38, www.jstor.org/stable/43609020.

13 *Girl juggle twelve hoops:* Spears, "Women's Sport in Ancient Greece," 39.

13 *Amazon rumors:* Adrienne Mayor, *The Amazons: Lives & Legends of Warrior Women Across the Ancient World* (Princeton, NJ: Princeton University Press, 2014): 84–94.

14 *Abandoned on a mountainside:* Mayor, *The Amazons,* 1.

14 *Beat her in a footrace:* Ovid, *Metamorphoses*, trans. Alexander Pope, John Dryden, Sir Samuel Garth, et al. (Pantianos Classics, 2016): 111–13.

15 *Scythian remains:* Mayor, *The Amazons,* 20, 29, 157.

15 *"If you think about it":* Simon Worrall, "Amazon Warriors Did Indeed Fight and Die like Men," *National Geographic,* October 28, 2014, https://www.nationalgeographic.com/news/2014/10/141029-amazons-scythians-hunger-games-herodotus-ice-princess-tattoo-cannabis.

15 *Amazon myth busting:* Worrall, "Amazon Warriors."

16 *"Both fascinated and appalled":* Worrall, "Amazon Warriors."

16 *"Yearning and desire":* Joshua Rothman, "The Real Amazons," *New Yorker,* October 17, 2014, https://www.newyorker.com/books/joshua-rothman/real-amazons.

17 *Villa Romana del Casale:* Mariella Radaelli, "The Bikini Girls, Archaeological Gems of Piazza Armerina," *L'Italo Americano,* May 18, 2017, https://italoamericano.org/story/2017-5-18/piazza-armerina.

18 *Playing sports in ancient Rome:* Carmello Bazzano, "Women and Sports in

Ancient Rome," *North American Society for Sports History Proceedings and Newsletter*, no. 6 (1977): 6.

18 *"For each vase":* Spears, "Women's Sport in Ancient Greece," 46.

CHAPTER 2

21 *Queen Victoria background:* Kate Williams, "Queen Victoria: the Woman Who Redefined Britain's Monarchy," *BBC*, accessed October 27, 2019, https://www.bbc.com/timelines/ztn34j6.

21 *Smelling salts:* "7 Things You (Probably) Didn't Know About Queen Victoria," *History Extra*, last modified May 24, 2019, https://www.historyextra.com/period/victorian/queen-victoria-facts-life-children-prince-albert-husband-marriage-reign/.

21 *Walk down a set of stairs: History Extra*, "7 Things."

22 *"Boss her about":* William Craig Hosch, "A Glimpse of Queen Victoria Through Her Journals," *Armstrong Undergraduate Journal of History* 4, no. 1 (April 2014), https://www.armstrong.edu/history-journal/history-journal-a-glimpse-of-queen-victoria-through-her-journals.

22 *More than a quarter:* Sue Macy, *Winning Ways: A Photohistory of American Women in Sports* (New York: Henry Holt and Company, 1996): 30.

22 *Pedestrianism background:* Matthew Algeo, *Pedestrianism: When Watching People Walk Was America's Favorite Spectator Sport* (Chicago: Chicago Review Press, 2014): 105–118.

23 *Ada Anderson's training:* Dahn Shaulis, "Pedestriennes: Newsworthy but Controversial Women in Sporting Entertainment," *Journal of Sport History* 26, no. 1 (Spring 1999): 35.

23 *1,000 half miles in 1,000 half hours: Baltimore American Commercial Advertiser*, May 16, 1880, 4.

23 *"The woman can never":* Harry Hall, *The Pedestriennes: America's Forgotten Superstars* (Indianapolis, IN: Dog Ear Publishing, 2014), 58, Kindle.

24 *Seven times just to get to a quarter mile:* Hall, *The Pedestriennes*, 3.

24 *As many as four thousand people:* "Not Yet Too Tired to Sing," *Sun* (New York), December 26, 1878, 1.

24 *Two dollars for reserved seating:* Algeo, *Pedestrianism*, 112.

24 *"The little hall":* "A Great Pedestrian Feat," *New York Times*, January 14, 1879, 5.

24 *"Largely composed of women":* "Still on the Track," *New York Times*, January 11, 1879, 5.

24 *Sealskin dresses and hats:* "Victorious," *Brooklyn Daily Eagle*, January 14, 1879, 3.

24 *In just 2:37.75:* "Madame Anderson's Plucky Walk," *Frank Leslie's Illustrated Newspaper*, February 1, 1879.

24 *Earned a cool $8,000:* Shaulis, "Mme. Anderson's Success," *New York Herald*, January 14, 1879, 8.

24 *Sipped port wine:* "A Long Walk," *Brooklyn Daily Eagle*, December 18, 1878, 4.

25 *"Overthrow of the mistaken notion":* "Madame Anderson and Her Critics," *Brooklyn Daily Eagle*, January 14, 1879, 2.

25 *"Slightly masculine":* Algeo, *Pedestrianism*, 109.

26 *Mark the faces of crowd members:* Hall, *The Pedestriennes*, 92.

26 *"Poetry of motion":* "Pedestrian Exercise for Women," *Brooklyn Daily Eagle*, December 29, 1878, 2.

26 *"Generally less graceful":* J. H. Kellogg, *Plain Facts for Old and Young* (Burlington, IA: Segner & Condit, 1881), 39–40.

26 *"Awkward" running gait:* Colette Dowling, *The Frailty Myth: Women Approaching Physical Equality* (New York: Random House, 2000), 17.

27 *Men were not allowed:* "Waterloo for Berkeley Girls, Stanford's Fair Basket Ball Players Won by a Goal," *San Francisco Examiner*, April 5, 1896, 11.

27 *Batted them away with sticks:* "The First Game," 125 Stanford Stories, accessed October 27, 2019, https://125.stanford.edu/the-first-game/.

27 *Naismith himself:* Mariah Burton Nelson, *The Stronger Women Get, the More Men Love Football: Sexism and the American Culture of Sports* (New York: Harcourt Brace, 1994), 14.

27 *"The fighting was hard":* "How the Game Went: The Merry Men of Both Teams Worked with a Will," *San Francisco Examiner*, April 5, 1896, 11.

28 *"Curly for the most part":* "Co-eds in Red Beat at Ball," *San Francisco Chronicle*, April 5, 1896, 26.

28 *"Missed the basket repeatedly:* "Co-eds in Red," *San Francisco Chronicle,* 26.

28 *Janitor and his assistant:* "Co-eds in Red," *San Francisco Chronicle,* 26.

28 *"In their dark blouses and bloomers":* Nelson, *The Stronger Women Get,* 14.

29 *"Grimy and generally disheveled":* Nelson, *The Stronger Women Get,* 14.

29 *Stanford had discontinued women's intercollegiate sports:* 125 Stanford Stories, "The First Game."

29 *Doctors, teachers, a nurse:* Sue Macy, *Basketball Belles: How Two Teams and One Scrappy Player Put Women's Hoops on the Map* (New York: Holiday House, 2011), "Author's Note," Adobe Digital Edition.

29 *Catharine Beecher:* Michael Sturges, "Catharine Beecher, Champion of Women's Education," last modified September 5, 2019, https://connecticuthistory.org/catharine-beecher-champion-of-womens-education/.

29 *"Confinement to one position":* Miss Catharine E. Beecher, *A Treatise on Domestic Economy, for the Use of Young Ladies at Home and at School* (Boston: Thomas H. Webb & Co., 1841), 12.

32 *"I could vault":* Charlotte Perkins Gilman, *The Living of Charlotte Perkins Gilman: An Autobiography* (Madison: The University of Wisconsin Press, 1990), 67.

32 *"Atalanta guidebook":* Patricia Vertinsky, "Feminist Charlotte Perkins Gilman's Pursuit of Health and Physical Fitness as a Strategy for Emancipation," *Journal of Sports History* 16, no. 1 (Spring 1989): 8, www.jstor.org/stable/43609379.

32 *"Spend life with":* William Blaikie, *How to Get Strong and How to Stay So* (New York: Harper & Brothers, 1879), 63.

32 *"Any muscle, well developed":* William Blaikie, *How to Get Strong and How to Stay So* (London: Sampson Low, Marston & Company, 1899), 34.

32 *"Happy to the verge of idiocy":* Vertinsky, "Charlotte Perkins Gilman's Pursuit of Health," 11.

32 *"She became very muscular!":* "The Wife and the Writer, Should Literary Women Be Addicted to the Marriage Habit?" *San Francisco Examiner,* December 19, 1892, 3.

32 American Farmer *magazine:* Macy, *Winning Ways,* 17.

33 *Tied her laces too tight:* Macy, *Winning Ways,* 18–19.

33 *"The boys were lucky":* Dowling, *The Frailty Myth*, 13.

33 *"Fresh air is absolutely essential":* Elisabeth Robinson Scovil, *Preparation for Motherhood* (Philadelphia: Henry Altemus, 1896), 39.

33 *Vassar College:* Macy, *Winning Ways*, 22.

34 *British Boxing Board of Control:* Neil Bennett, "Round One for Women's Boxing," BBC News, November 24, 1998, http://news.bbc.co.uk/2/hi/sport/218581.stm.

34 *Fu Yuanhui:* Emily Fend, "Uninhibited Chinese Swimmer, Discussing Her Period, Shatters Another Barrier," *New York Times*, August 16, 2016, https://www.nytimes.com/2016/08/17/world/asia/china-fu-yuanhui-period-olympics.html.

34 *The "great woman revolution":* Mary F. Eastman, *The Biography of Dr. Dio Lewis* (New York: Fowler & Wells Co., 1891), 122.

34 *Boys and girls should exercise together:* Dio Lewis, "The New Gymnastics," *Atlantic*, August 1862, https://www.theatlantic.com/magazine/archive/1862/08/the-new-gymnastics/305408/.

34 *"Girls do not really step on the ground":* Dr. Dio Lewis, *Our Girls* (New York: Harper & Brothers, 1871), 22–23.

35 *"Black velvet knee breeches":* "A Long Walk," 4.

36 *"Femininity principle":* "Rules of Conduct," AAGPBL Rules of Conduct, accessed October 27, 2019, https://www.aagpbl.org/history/rules-of-conduct.

37 *"The woman's desire":* Dr. Silas Weir Mitchell, *Doctor and Patient* (Philadelphia: J. B. Lippincott Company, 1888), 2.

38 *"Not* made *for governing":* Queen Victoria, *The Letters of Queen Victoria*, ed. A. C. Benson, Reginald Brett, and Viscount Esther (Cambridge: Cambridge University Press, 2014), 438.

38 *"Her physical powers": Brooklyn Daily Eagle*, "Pedestrian Exercise for Women," 2.

38 *"First began my walk":* "Singing While She Walks," *Sun* (New York), December 31, 1878, 3.

CHAPTER 3

41 *Second only to September 11:* Valerie Wingfield, "The General Slocum Disaster of June 15, 1904," New York Public Library blog, June 13, 2011, https://www.nypl.org/blog/2011/06/13/great-slocum-disaster-june-15-1904.

41 *Seven to ten yards of fabric:* Marilyn Morgan, "Bodysuits & Boots: Early Swimsuits for Women," ConsumingCultures.net, March 13, 2017, http://www.consumingcultures.net/2017/03/13/bodysuits-boots-early-swimsuits-for-women/.

42 *Wool and flannel were the recommended:* Morgan, "Bodysuits & Boots."

42 *Kids went for free:* "1,000 Lives May Be Lost in Burning of the Excursion Boat Gen. Slocum," *New York Times*, June 16, 1904, 1.

42 *"Like trying to put out hell itself":* Gilbert King, "A Spectacle of Horror—The Burning of the General Slocum," Smithsonian.com, February 21, 2012, https://www.smithsonianmag.com/history/a-spectacle-of-horror-the-burning-of-the-general-slocum-104712974/.

42 *Flammable paint:* Edward T. O'Donnell, "The Dreadful End of Little Germany," *Spiegel*, April 7, 2006, https://www.spiegel.de/international/a-forgotten-new-york-disaster-the-dreadful-end-of-little-germany-a-410321.html.

42 *Captain fanned the flames:* King, "A Spectacle of Horror."

42 *Lifeboats were inaccessible:* Tim Higgins, "Easton Artist Captures Vision of 100-Year-Old New York City Tragedy in Paintings," *Morning Call*, January 5, 2018, https://www.mcall.com/entertainment/arts-theater/mc-ent-general-slocum-disaster-easton-cindy-vogjnovic-20171222-story.html.

42 *Crew had never practiced a fire drill:* King, "A Spectacle of Horror."

42 *Safety equipment crumbled:* King, "A Spectacle of Horror."

42 *Life jackets failed: New York Times*, "1,000 Lives May Be Lost," 1.

42 *"With sure death": New York Times*, "1,000 Lives May Be Lost," 1.

43 *321 survivors:* Wingfield, "The General Slocum Disaster."

43 *Aftermath of disaster:* Marilyn Morgan, "Drowning in Culture: Women & Swimming in the 20th Century US," ArchivesPublicHistory.org, March 22, 2017, http://www.archivespublichistory.org/?p=1645.

43 *"Practical and rational point of view":* Edwyn Sandys, "Swimming," in *Athletics and Out-door Sports for Women: Each Subject Being Separately Treated by a Special Writer*, ed. Lucille Eaton Hill (New York: The MacMillan Company, 1903), 97.

43 *"Not until then":* Edwyn Sandys, "Swimming," 97–98.

44 *Annette Kellermann's childhood:* Justin Parkinson, "Annette Kellerman: Hollywood's First Nude Star," *BBC News Magazine*, February 20, 2016, https://www.bbc.com/news/magazine-35472490.

44 *English Channel attempt:* Marilyn Morgan, "The 'Million Dollar Mermaid' Revolutionizes Women's Swimwear," ConsumingCultures.net, March 10, 2017, http://www.consumingcultures.net/2017/03/10/the-million-dollar-mermaid-revolutionizes-womens-swimwear/.

44 *Creating the one-piece bodysuit:* Parkinson, "Hollywood's First Nude Star."

45 *"I am certain":* Annette Kellermann, *How to Swim* (New York: George H. Doran Company, 1918), 47.

45 *Multiple manufacturers:* Kathleen Drowne and Patrick Huber, *The 1920s* (Westport, CT: Greenwood Press, 2004), 103.

45 *"Vitality, health, magnetism, and symmetry":* Hadley Meares, "This 'Million Dollar Mermaid' Urged Women to Be Physically Free," *Good*, April 16, 2018, https://www.good.is/articles/annette-kellerman.

45 *Cold cream slathered:* Meares, "Million Dollar Mermaid."

45 *"You cannot be brave":* Emily Gibson with Barbara Firth, *The Original Million Dollar Mermaid: The Annette Kellerman Story* (Sydney: Allen & Unwin, 2005), 88.

45 *Shocking step of disrobing:* Meares, "Million Dollar Mermaid."

45 *"Women are especially well fitted":* Annette Kellermann, "Swimming—Woman's Ideal Sport," *Physical Culture*, unknown date, 56.

48 *Pitonof wins Boston Light Swim:* Marjorie Ingall, "Remembering Rose Pitonof: The Real Coney Island Mermaid," *Tablet*, September 14, 2018, https://www.tabletmag.com/scroll/270822/remembering-rose-pitonof-the-real-coney-island-mermaid.

48 *"She was just a teenager":* Jaimie Monahan, interview with author, March 5, 2019.

48 *Claimed to have been arrested:* Kristin Toussaint, "This Woman's One-Piece Bathing Suit Got Her Arrested in 1907," Boston.com, July 2, 2015, https://www.boston.com/news/history/2015/07/02/this-womans-one-piece-bathing-suit-got-her-arrested-in-1907.

48 *"I can't swim":* "A Brief and Incomplete History of the Swimsuit," *Mental Floss,* May 29, 2015, http://mentalfloss.com/article/57024/brief-and-incomplete-history-swimsuit.

48 *"Modesty hood":* Karen Karbo, "From Gold Spangles to Gold Medals," in *Nike Is a Goddess,* ed. Lissa Smith (New York: Atlantic Monthly Press, 1998), 183.

48 *Clarendon Beach:* Drowne and Huber, *The 1920s,* 104.

48 *"First female swimmers":* Karbo, "From Gold Spangles to Gold Medals," 182.

49 *"Like a person":* Maureen Corrigan, "In Ederle Bio, a Channel-Crosser's Defiant Spirit," *NPR,* July 23, 2009, https://www.npr.org/templates/story/story.php?storyId=106857551.

49 *Olive oil, lanolin, petroleum jelly, and lard:* Kelli Anderson, "The Young Woman and the Sea," *Sports Illustrated,* November 29, 1999, 92.

49 *Fourteen extra miles:* Anderson, "The Young Woman and the Sea," 92.

49 *Ticker-tape parade:* Anderson, "The Young Woman and the Sea," 90, 92.

49 *British immigrations officer:* Noah Tesch, "8 Incredible Swimming Feats," accessed October 27, 2019, https://www.britannica.com/list/8-incredible-swimming-feats.

49 *"Even the most uncompromising champion":* John McCain with Mark Salter, *Hard Call: Great Decisions and the Extraordinary People Who Made Them* (New York: Twelve, 2007), 361, OverDrive.

49 *"Women have been shackled":* Dowling, *The Frailty Myth,* 6.

50 *"Positive predictor of life span"*: Greg Nuckols, interview with author, May 7, 2019.

50 *Men are still more likely to know how to swim:* International Life Saving Federation, "Drowning Facts and Figures," ILSF.org, https://www.ilsf.org/drowning-facts-and-figures/.

50 *Holds true even in U.S.:* American Red Cross, "Red Cross Launches Campaign to Cut Drowning in Half in 50 Cities," RedCross.org, May 20, 2014, https:

//www.redcross.org/about-us/news-and-events/press-release/red-cross-launches-campaign-to-cut-drowning-in-half-in-50-cities.html.

50 *Girls fill more of the ranks of competitive swimmers:* Paul Steinbach, "More Females Still Swim and Dive, but Males Narrowing the Gap," *Athletic Business,* November 2007, https://www.athleticbusiness.com/Aquatics/more-females-still-swim-and-dive-but-males-narrowing-the-gap.html and Daniel D'Addona, "High School Swimming and Diving Grows to 138,935 Participants," *Swimming World,* September 12, 2018, https://www.swimmingworldmagazine.com/news/high-school-swimming-and-diving-grows-to-138935-participants/.

50 *Recent tsunamis:* Lori M. Hunter, Joan Castro, Danika Kleiber, and Kendra Hutchens, "Swimming and Gendered Vulnerabilities: Evidence from the Northern and Central Philippines," *Society & Natural Resources* 29, no. 3 (2016): 380–85, https://www.ncbi.nlm.nih.gov/pmc/articles/PMC4835034/.

CHAPTER 4

53 *Circus background: The Circus: Part I,* directed by Sharon Grimberg, PBS, October 9, 2018.

53 *Katharina Brumbach's birth:* Jan Todd, "Center Ring: Katie Sandwina and the Construction of Celebrity," *Iron Game History,* November 2007, 8.

54 *"Put a half-dollar":* John D. Fair, "Kati Sandwina: 'Hercules Can Be a Lady,'" *Iron Game History,* December 2005, 5.

54 *Fifteen-inch biceps:* Debbie Foulkes, "Katie Sandwina (1884–1952): Circus Strongwoman," ForgottenNewsmakers.com, December 14, 2010, https://forgottennewsmakers.com/2010/12/14/katie-sandwina-1884-%e2%80%93-1952-circus-strongwoman/.

54 *Handstands at age two:* Todd, "Center Ring," 8.

54 *Lifting in adolescence:* Foulkes, "Katie Sandwina."

54 *One hundred German marks:* Foulkes, "Katie Sandwina."

54 *Fell in love:* Tessa Hulls, "The Great Sandwina, Circus Strongwoman and Restaurateur," *Atlas Obscura,* December 26, 2017, https://www.atlasobscura.com/articles/the-great-sandwina.

54 *1902 showdown with Sandow:* Hulls, "The Great Sandwina."

54 *Wrestled a muzzled lion:* Conor Heffernan, "Sandow the Lion Tamer," PhysicalCultureStudy.com, August 18, 2016.

54 *"Something to lift, throw, or project":* David L. Chapman and Patricia Vertinsky, *Venus with Biceps: A Pictorial History of Muscular Women* (Vancouver: Arsenal Pulp Press, 2010), 130.

55 *Siegmund Breitbart:* Fair, "Hercules Can Be a Lady," 4.

55 *"A little light housework":* Kate Carew, "Barnum and Bailey's 'Strong Woman' Tells Kate Carew—This Young Goddess of the Tan-Bark, Who Tosses Her Husband About as She Would a Feather, Explains How She Came by Her Strength," *San Francisco Examiner*, April 30, 1911, 79.

55 *Performed in two shows:* Todd, "Center Ring," 7.

55 *50 pounds by the age of two:* Todd, "Center Ring," 7.

55 *Dumbbell as a toy:* Todd, "Center Ring," 7.

55 *Breaking a Bulldog chain:* Robert Nealey, "The Feminine Sandow: Katie Sandwina," *IronMan*, January 1961, 20–21, 46–47.

56 *"The feminine Hercules":* Todd, "Center Ring," 10.

56 *"Panther-like":* Marguerite Martyn, " 'The Lady Hercules' Tells Marguerite Martyn," *St. Louis Post-Dispatch*, June 4, 1911, 1B.

57 *"A totalizing nomadic circus":* Janet M. Davis, interview with author, May 16, 2019.

57 *"Within the show grounds":* Davis, interview with author.

58 *Up to $1,500 a week:* Fair, "Hercules Can Be a Lady," 4.

58 *Athleta, who could waltz:* Jan Todd, "Bring on the Amazons: An Evolutionary History," in *Picturing the Modern Amazon*, ed. Joanna Frueh, Laurie Fierstein, and Judith Stein (New York: Rizzoli, 2000).

58 *Crab position with a seesaw:* Chapman and Vertinsky, *Venus with Biceps*, 65.

58 *Stopped a runaway horse . . . and freed a wagon:* David P. Webster, "The Atlas & Vulcana Group of Society Athletes," *Iron Game History*, May/June 2000, 28.

58 *"When you hear or read":* E. K. and L. M. Reader, "Types of Women Athletes," *Sandow's Magazine of Physical Culture*, date unknown, 252.

58 *Minerva's lifts:* Jan Todd, "The Mystery of Minerva," *Iron Game History*, April 1990, 15.

59 *Lifted eighteen men:* Chapman and Vertinsky, *Venus with Biceps*, 33.

59 *"Principal part of my existence":* Todd, "The Mystery of Minerva," 15.

59 *"Women become the focal point":* Davis, interview with author.

59 *Outspoken equestrian performers:* Kat Vecchio, "Barnum & Bailey's Forgotten High-Flying Suffragists," *Narratively*, December 27, 2017, https://narratively.com/barnum-bailey-forgotten-high-flying-suffragists/.

59 *"There is no class of women":* Vecchio, "High-Flying Suffragists."

60 *"If physical strength":* Martyn, " 'The Lady Hercules' Tells Marguerite Martyn," 1B.

60 *Vice president:* Hulls, "The Great Sandwina."

60 *"Tremble for the future of the anti-cause":* Todd, "Center Ring," 7.

60 *"You earn salaries":* Vecchio, "High-Flying Suffragists."

60 *Circus man barged into:* Vecchio, "High-Flying Suffragists."

61 *Two million bikes sold in 1897:* Peter Zheutlin, "Women on Wheels: The Bicycle and the Women's Movement of the 1890s," AnnieLondonderry.com, accessed October 26, 2019, http://www.annielondonderry.com/womenWheels.html.

61 *Estimated 2 million American women:* Gary Kamiya, "Sex and Cycling: How Bike Craze Aroused Passions in 1890s San Francisco," *San Francisco Chronicle*, October 18, 2019, https://www.sfchronicle.com/bayarea/article/Sex-and-cycling-How-bike-craze-aroused-passions-14544576.php.

61 *Until her sixteenth birthday:* Frances E. Willard, *A Wheel Within a Wheel: How I Learned to Ride the Bicycle, with Some Reflections by the Way* (New York: Fleming H. Revell Company, 1895), 9–10.

61 *"In my heart of hearts":* Willard, *A Wheel Within a Wheel*, 10.

61 *"I remember writing in my journal":* Willard, *A Wheel Within a Wheel*, 10.

62 *"Beloved and breezy outdoor world":* Willard, *A Wheel Within a Wheel*, 10.

62 *Three months of practicing:* Willard, *A Wheel Within a Wheel*, 74.

62 *Gladys:* Frances Willard House Museum and Archives, "Collections Object – Willard's Bicycle," FrancesWillardHouse.org, November 12, 2015, https://franceswillardhouse.org/gladys-the-bicycle/.

62 *"Less than a single day":* Willard, *A Wheel Within a Wheel*, 75.

63 *"Myself plus the bicycle":* Willard, *A Wheel Within a Wheel*, 27–28.

63 *"Deliverance, revolution, salvation":* Mrs. Reginald de Koven, "Bicycling for Women," *Cosmopolitan*, August 1895.

63 *Many physicians were supportive:* Nelson, *The Stronger Women Get*, 16.

63 *"If women ride":* Willard, *A Wheel Within a Wheel*, 39–40.

64 *Bicycle critics:* Mariah Burton Nelson, "Introduction," in *Nike Is a Goddess*, ed. Lissa Smith (New York: Atlantic Monthly Press, 1998), xiv.

64 *Invited lewd commentary:* Nelson, *The Stronger Women Get*, 16.

64 *Bicycle face:* Joseph Stromberg, "'Bicycle Face': a 19th-Century Health Problem Made Up to Scare Women away from Biking," *Vox*, March 24, 2015, https://www.vox.com/2014/7/8/5880931/the-19th-century-health-scare-that-told-women-to-worry-about-bicycle.

64 *"Most vicious thing":* "Bab in Washington," *Sunday Herald*, July 19, 1891, 9.

64 *Suffragists blocked Winston Churchill's motorcade:* JR Thorpe, "The Feminist History of Bicycles," *Bustle*, May 12, 2017, https://www.bustle.com/p/the-feminist-history-of-bicycles-57455.

64 *New Woman . . . on a bicycle:* Kenna Howat, "Pedaling the Path to Freedom: American Women on Bicycles," National Women's History Museum, June 27, 2017, https://www.womenshistory.org/articles/pedaling-path-freedom.

65 *Von Hillern hats and photos:* Shaulis, "Pedestriennes," 34.

65 *"Apostle of muscular religion":* Shaulis, "Pedestriennes," 34.

65 *"Though women may not practice":* "A Defeat and a Triumph," *New York Times*, November 18, 1876, 4.

65 *"In her presence":* Carew, "Barnum and Bailey's 'Strong Woman,'" 79.

CHAPTER 5

68 *Kate Giroux came up with an idea:* Harold Zinkin with Bonnie Hearn, *Remembering Muscle Beach: Where Hard Bodies Began* (Santa Monica, CA: Angel City Press, 1999): 17–18.

68 *Mussel Beach:* Steve Harvey, "Mussel or Muscle: Whatever You Call It, It's a Beach That's Not Forgotten by Its Many Devotees," *Los Angeles Times*,

March 30, 1986, https://www.latimes.com/archives/la-xpm-1986-03-30-me-1736-story.html.

68 *Santa Monica added:* Danny, "History of Muscle Beach (Part 1)," TheIronWitness.com, April 3, 2016, http://theironwitness.com/muscle-beach-history-part-1/.

68 *Hamburgers and five-cent ice cream:* Article in *Muscular Development,* unknown author, title, and date, Abbye (Pudgy) and Les Stockton Papers, H. J. Lutcher Stark Center for Physical Culture & Sports, University of Texas at Austin.

68 *Jukeboxes blasted:* Zinkin, *Remembering Muscle Beach,* 17.

69 *"Called us 'Muscleheads'":* Zinkin, *Remembering Muscle Beach,* 14.

69 *On a per-square-foot basis:* Zinkin, *Remembering Muscle Beach,* 15.

69 *Abby Eville background:* Jan Todd, "The Legacy of Pudgy Stockton," *Iron Game History,* January 1992, 5–6.

69 *Bob Hoffman:* Todd, "The Legacy of Pudgy Stockton," 5.

70 *Reluctant at first:* Marla Matzer Rose, *Muscle Beach: Where the Best Bodies in the World Started a Fitness Revolution* (New York: LA Weekly Books, 2001), 49.

70 *Main turning point:* Wayne Wilson and David K. Wiggins, editors, *LA Sports: Play, Games, and Community in the City of Angels* (Fayetteville, AR: University of Arkansas Press, 2018), 248.

71 *"Pudgy and her boys":* Todd, "The Legacy of Pudgy Stockton," 6.

71 *More than forty magazines:* Todd, "The Legacy of Pudgy Stockton," 6.

71 *"Gigantic and beautiful":* Carew, "Barnum and Bailey's 'Strong Woman,'" 79.

71 *200-pound anvil:* Fair, "Hercules Can Be a Lady," 6.

71 *"New type of woman":* Todd, "The Legacy of Pudgy Stockton," 5.

72 *Edna Rivers:* Pudgy Stockton, "Barbelles," *Strength and Health,* no month available, 1944, 11, Abbye (Pudgy) and Les Stockton Papers, H. J. Lutcher Stark Center for Physical Culture & Sports, University of Texas at Austin.

72 *Kay Brougham:* Pudgy Stockton, "Barbelles," *Strength and Health,* no month available, 1945, no page number available, Abbye (Pudgy) and Les Stockton Papers, H. J. Lutcher Stark Center for Physical Culture & Sports, University of Texas at Austin.

72 *Bowling shoes for lifting:* Pudgy Stockton, "Barbelles," *Strength and Health,*

no month available, 1944, no page number available, Abbye (Pudgy) and Les Stockton Papers, H. J. Lutcher Stark Center for Physical Culture & Sports, University of Texas at Austin.

72 *"Dissipating pleasures":* Pudgy Stockton, "Barbelles," *Strength and Health,* no month available, 1946, 45, Abbye (Pudgy) and Les Stockton Papers, H. J. Lutcher Stark Center for Physical Culture & Sports, University of Texas at Austin.

73 *Maureen O'Brien:* Pudgy Stockton, "Barbelles," *Strength and Health,* no month available, 1944, 39, Abbye (Pudgy) and Les Stockton Papers, H. J. Lutcher Stark Center for Physical Culture & Sports, University of Texas at Austin.

73 *"Queer looks":* Margaret Smith, letter to Pudgy Stockton, May 1, 1954, Abbye (Pudgy) and Les Stockton Papers, H. J. Lutcher Stark Center for Physical Culture & Sports, University of Texas at Austin.

73 *"Carrot on the stick":* Al Thomas, "Out of the Past . . . a Fond Remembrance: Abbye 'Pudgy' Stockton," *Body and Power,* March 1983, 10.

73 *"One afternoon I wandered":* Thomas, "Out of the Past," 14–15.

74 *Muscle Beach Weightlifting Club:* Danny, "History of Muscle Beach."

74 *First woman to garner attention:* Wilson and Wiggins, *LA Sports,* 249.

74 *Burned by boiling water:* Zinkin, *Remembering Muscle Beach,* 51.

74 *Bending iron bars and walking on wires:* Wilson and Wiggins, *LA Sports,* 249.

74 *Relished the attention:* Wilson and Wiggins, *LA Sports,* 249.

74 *Los Angeles phone book:* Sue Macy, "Finding Relna," I. N. K.: Interesting Nonfiction for Kids blog, July 2, 2009, http://inkrethink.blogspot.com/2009/07/finding-relna.html.

74 *Decoy for Marilyn Monroe:* Macy, "Finding Relna."

74 *Fifty major newspapers:* Jan Todd, "Picturing Amazons: Journalism and Muscular Womanhood," *Proceedings of the North American Society for Sport History,* 1998: 20.

75 *"Fake, fake":* Zinkin, *Remembering Muscle Beach,* 53.

75 *Thirty-five handstand press-ups:* Jan Todd, "Growing Up Strong: Pat McCormick, Relna Brewer and Muscle Beach," *Proceedings of the North American Society for Sport History,* 2001, 109.

75 *Cannonballs:* Karen Rosen, "Olympic Champ Pat McCormick Still Up to Her Old Tricks," TeamUSA.org, October 5, 2012, https://www.teamusa.org/News/2012/October/15/Olympic-Champ-Pat-McCormick-Still-Up-To-Her-Old-Tricks.

75 *"At age 10":* LA84 Foundation, "An Olympian's Oral History: Pat McCormick," Margaret Costa interviewing Pat McCormick, July 26, 1991, 2, https://digital.la84.org/digital/collection/p17103coll11/id/222/.

75 *Bigger font:* Harvey, "Mussel or Muscle."

78 *"An uninformed nation":* Zinkin, *Remembering Muscle Beach,* 126.

78 *Salads and raw milk:* Harvey, "Mussel or Muscle."

78 *"Every time you came down": California's Gold,* "Muscle Beach," hosted by Huell Howser, aired 1999 on KCET Los Angeles.

78 *"I remember this camaraderie":* Randy Boelsems, interview with author, May 14, 2019.

78 *"The girls, flying through the air":* Les Stockton, letter to Bonnie Hearn, December 16, 1998, Abbye (Pudgy) and Les Stockton Papers, H. J. Lutcher Stark Center for Physical Culture & Sports, University of Texas at Austin.

79 *"The most important thing":* Zinkin, *Remembering Muscle Beach,* 125.

79 *"The grief grind":* Tina Plakinger, "The Legacy of Muscle Beach," *IronMan,* July 1992, 146.

79 *First sanctioned weightlifting competition:* Todd, "The Legacy of Pudgy Stockton," 7.

79 *Women's-only health club:* Elena Conis, "A 'Lady of Iron' and a Model for Fitness," *Los Angeles Times,* January 7, 2008, https://www.latimes.com/archives/la-xpm-2008-jan-07-he-esoterica7-story.html.

79 *"Every woman bodybuilder":* Todd, "The Legacy of Pudgy Stockton," 7.

80 *"When I first started":* Carol Ann Weber, "Happy Ever Aftering in California Camelot—Muscle Beach," *Beach News & Entertainment,* June 1996, 7.

80 *"In the 40's era":* Les Stockton, letter to Joe Roark, November 7, 1988, Abbye (Pudgy) and Les Stockton Papers, H. J. Lutcher Stark Center for Physical Culture & Sports, University of Texas at Austin.

CHAPTER 6

83 *Sewed gunnysacks:* "Babe Didrikson Zaharias," Encyclopedia.com, last modified September 19, 2019, https://www.encyclopedia.com/people/sports-and-games/sports-biographies/babe-didrikson-zaharias.

83 *Running around barefoot:* Roseanne Montillo, *Fire on the Track: Betty Robinson and the Triumph of the Early Olympic Women* (New York: Crown, 2017), 92.

83 *Girls' hobbies boring:* Don Van Natta Jr., *Wonder Girl: The Magnificent Sporting Life of Babe Didrikson Zaharias* (New York: Little, Brown and Company, 2011), 58, OverDrive.

83 *Repeated a grade:* Van Natta Jr., *Wonder Girl,* 71.

83 *Dropped out:* Evan Andrews, "10 Things You May Not Know About Babe Didrikson Zaharias," History.com, last updated August 22, 2018, https://www.history.com/news/10-things-you-may-not-know-about-babe-didrikson-zaharias.

84 *"Is Babe Didrikson the greatest?":* Jimmy Jemail, "The Question: Is Babe Didrikson the Greatest All-Round Athlete of All Time?," *Sports Illustrated,* June 6, 1955, 6–7.

84 *Miscellaneous:* Larry Schwartz, "Didrikson Was a Woman Ahead of Her Time," ESPN.com, accessed October 22, 2019, https://www.espn.com/sportscentury/features/00014147.html.

84 *"Dolls":* Schwartz, "Ahead of Her Time."

84 *1932 AAU meet:* Van Natta Jr., "Wonder Girl," 122–42.

85 *Running, jumping,* and *throwing:* Andrews, "10 Things You May Not Know."

85 *Vaudeville circuit:* "Remembering a 'Babe' Sports Fans Shouldn't Forget," *NPR,* June 6, 2011, https://www.npr.org/2011/06/26/137319975/remembering-a-babe-sports-fans-shouldnt-forget.

85 *"Hard-bitten":* Paul Gallico, *Farewell to Sport* (New York: Alfred A. Knopf, 1938), 239.

86 *"Waited for the phone to ring":* Schwartz, "Ahead of Her Time."

86 *Joe DiMaggio:* Encyclopedia.com, "Babe Didrikson Zaharias."

86 *Bras and girdles:* Jon Henderson, "Babe Didrikson, the Greatest Female Ath-

lete of All Time?," *The Guardian*, October 2, 2006, https://www.theguardian.com/sport/blog/2006/oct/02/babedidriksonthegreatestfe.

86 *Who was playing for second:* David Barron, "Best Female Athlete? No One's Ever Beaten Babe," *Houston Chronicle*, July 29, 2013, https://www.houstonchronicle.com/news/article/Best-female-athlete-No-one-s-ever-beaten-Babe-4694572.php.

87 *Nature of their relationship:* Van Natta Jr., "Wonder Girl," 601–02.

87 *$2 million in endorsements:* Jim Buzinski, "Moment #3: Tennis Great Billie Jean King Outed," Outsports.com, October 2, 2011, https://www.outsports.com/2011/10/2/4051938/moment-3-tennis-great-billie-jean-king-outed.

87 *46 percent of women:* "Empowering Women in Sports: Barriers to Women in Athletic Careers," Feminist Majority Foundation, accessed October 23, 2019, https://www.feminist.org/research/sports/sports4.html.

87 *"The cliché that exists":* Kate Fagan, "After the Storm," *espnW*, October 4, 2014, http://www.espn.com/espn/feature/story/_/id/11655083/us-women-soccer-star-abby-wambach-lives-extreme.

87 *"Girls in sports":* "Do You Know the Factors Influencing Girls' Participation in Sports?," Women's Sports Foundation, accessed October 23, 2019, https://www.womenssportsfoundation.org/do-you-know-the-factors-influencing-girls-participation-in-sports.

88 *Brittney Griner and Jason Collins:* Jonathan Zimmerman, "The Double Standard of Sports Sexuality," *Globe and Mail*, May 1, 2013, https://www.theglobeandmail.com/opinion/the-double-standard-of-sports-sexuality/article11642057.

88 *"Call it the double standard":* Zimmerman, "The Double Standard."

88 *68 percent of high school seniors:* "Play to Win: Improving the Lives of LGBTQ Youth in Sports," Human Rights Campaign Foundation, 2018, 7.

88 *"Across our society":* Zimmerman, "The Double Standard."

88 *"Babe Is a Lady Now":* Gene Farmer, "What a Babe!," *Life*, June 23, 1947, 90.

89 *Bigger breasts:* Pete Martin, "Babe Didrikson Takes Off Her Mask," *Saturday Evening Post*, September 20, 1947, 26.

89 *Six feet tall and 225 pounds:* William Oscar Johnson and Nancy Williamson, "Babe Part 2," *Sports Illustrated*, October 13, 1975, 57.

89 *"No matter how good they are":* Gallico, *Farewell to Sport,* 244.

89 *"Handsome young girls":* Gallico, *Farewell to Sport,* 246.

89 *Ugly duckling:* Gallico, *Farewell to Sport,* 240.

89 *"Man-snatching":* Gallico, *Farewell to Sport,* 239.

89 *"Splendid woman":* Paul Gallico, *The Golden People* (Garden City, NY: Doubleday & Company, 1965), 237.

89 *"Transition from the man-girl":* Gallico, *The Golden People,* 248.

89 *Lost a golf match and a footrace:* Van Natta Jr., "Wonder Girl," 178–81.

89 *"Great big he-man":* Dave Zirin, *Game Over: How Politics Has Turned the Sports World Upside Down* (New York: The New Press, 2013), 145.

90 *"People used to say":* "Abbye Stockton, 88, Weight-Lifting Pioneer, Dies," *New York Times,* July 10, 2006, https://www.nytimes.com/2006/07/10/sports/10stockton.html.

91 *"Maybe having a baby":* Rob Haskell, "Serena Williams on Motherhood, Marriage, and Making Her Comeback," *Vogue,* January 10, 2018, https://www.vogue.com/article/serena-williams-vogue-cover-interview-february-2018.

91 *Randall was the only mom:* "2018 U.S. Olympic Team Fun Facts," TeamUSA.org, accessed October 23, 2019, https://www.teamusa.org/PyeongChang-2018-Olympic-Winter-Games/Team-USA/Fun-Facts.

91 *Team USA mothers and fathers:* TeamUSA.org, "2018 Fun Facts."

91 *"A bigger toll":* Caroline Bologna, "Team USA's Only Mom Athlete Opens Up About Parenthood," HuffPost.com, February 11, 2018, https://www.huffpost.com/entry/kikkan-randall-olympics-mother_n_5a786943e4b0905433b6bae3.

92 *Five dropped out . . . five collapsed:* Roger Robinson, "Eleven Wretched Women," *Running Times,* May 14, 2012, https://www.runnersworld.com/advanced/a20802639/eleven-wretched-women/.

92 *"Not a very edifying spectacle":* Knute K. Rockne, "Yankees Have Another Dull Day in Olympics," *Pittsburgh Press,* August 3, 1928, 32.

92 *"Too great a call":* Jeré Longman, "How the Women Won," *New York Times,* June 23, 1996, https://www.nytimes.com/1996/06/23/magazine/how-the-women-won.html.

92 *"220-yard dash is long enough":* Montillo, *Fire on the Track,* 89.

93 *What really happened in the 800-meter race:* Robinson, "Eleven Wretched Women," and Colleen English, "Not a Very Edifying Spectacle": The Controversial Women's 800-Meter Race in the 1928 Olympics," *Sport in American History,* October 8, 2015, https://ussporthistory.com/2015/10/08/not-a-very-edifying-spectacle-the-controversial-womens-800-meter-race-in-the-1928-olympics/.

93 *Men's 800 meters in 1904:* "Americans Make More Records at Stadium," *St. Louis Globe-Democrat,* September 2, 1904, 6.

94 *"The accusations followed":* Montillo, *Fire on the Track,* 235.

94 *Avery Brundage certifying womanhood:* Erin E. Buzuvis, "Hormone Check: Critique of Olympic Rules on Sex and Gender," *Wisconsin Journal of Law, Gender & Society* 31, no. 1 (2016): 29–56.

94 *"You know, the ancient Greeks":* Roger Butterfield, "Avery Brundage," *Life,* June 14, 1948, 120.

94 *Underwear, and ran them up a flagpole:* Rosen, "Olympic Champ Pat McCormick."

95 *Invasive test:* Dean Eastmond, "Caster Semenya's Problem Isn't That She's Intersex—It's That Her Femininity Doesn't Look How We Want It To," *Independent,* August 22, 2016, https://www.independent.co.uk/voices/caster-semenya-rio-2016-gold-800m-intersex-gender-femininity-doesnt-look-the-way-we-want-a7203506.html.

95 *Court of Arbitration for Sport:* Jeré Longman and Juliet Macur, "Caster Semenya Loses Case to Compete as a Woman in All Races," *New York Times,* May 1, 2019, https://www.nytimes.com/2019/05/01/sports/caster-semenya-loses.html.

95 *Meet record in Doha:* Sean Ingle, "Caster Semenya Wins 800m in Doha and Fends Off Retirement Talk," *Guardian,* May 3, 2019, https://www.theguardian.com/sport/2019/may/03/caster-semenya-wins-800m-doha-diamond-league-case-iaaf-athletics.

95 *"Loving one another":* Eastmond, "Caster Semenya's Problem."

95 *History of proving womanhood:* Vanessa Heggie, "Testing Sex and Gender in Sports; Reinventing, Reimagining and Reconstructing Histories," *Endeavour* 34, no. 4 (December 2010): 157–63.

96 *Dora Ratjen:* Mike Henson, "Sex and Gender in Hitler's Shadow: Dora Ratjen and the 1936 Olympics," *Vice,* August 11, 2016, https://www.vice.com/en_us

/article/qkyvym/sex-and-gender-in-hitlers-shadow-dora-ratjen-and-the-1936-olympics.

96 *No good evidence that he competed fraudulently:* Heggie, "Testing Sex and Gender in Sports," 157–63.

96 *Soccer goalie in Texas:* Gary Libman, "Kicking Up a Storm," *Los Angeles Times,* November 8, 1990, E1, E14, E15.

97 *"In other words":* Daniel Engber, "Should Caster Semenya Be Allowed to Compete Against Women?," *Slate,* August 5, 2016, https://slate.com/culture/2016/08/should-caster-semenya-be-allowed-to-compete-against-women.html.

97 *Testosterone's advantage:* Gina Kolata, "Does Testosterone Really Give Caster Semenya an Edge on the Track?" *New York Times,* May 1, 2019, https://www.nytimes.com/2019/05/01/health/caster-semenya-testosterone.html.

98 *Prank phone calls:* Van Natta Jr., "Wonder Girl," 396.

98 *"Let me tell you girls something":* Van Natta Jr., "Wonder Girl," 402.

99 *"An incredible human being":* Johnson and Williamson, "Babe Part 2," 49.

CHAPTER 7

102 *"Give me those numbers":* Sarah Lorge Butler, "How Kathrine Switzer Paved the Way," *espnW,* April 11, 2012, https://www.espn.com/espnw/news-commentary/story/_/id/7803502/2012-boston-marathon-how-kathrine-switzer-paved-way-female-runners.

102 *Circumvent the rules:* Andy Frye, "Kathrine Switzer Talks Marathon, 1967 and Now," Forbes.com, April 2, 2019, https://www.forbes.com/sites/andyfrye/2019/04/02/kathrine-switzer-talks-boston-marathon/#3881f876a35d.

102 *Using initials:* Frye, "Kathrine Switzer Talks Marathon."

103 *Bobbi Gibb:* Ailsa Ross, "The Woman Who Crashed the Boston Marathon," *JSTOR Daily,* March 18, 2018, https://daily.jstor.org/the-woman-who-crashed-the-boston-marathon/.

103 *Plenty of skepticism:* Kathrine Switzer, "The Real Story," KathrineSwitzer.com, accessed October 23, 2019, https://kathrineswitzer.com/1967-boston-marathon-the-real-story/.

103 *"Women were deemed fragile":* Kathrine Switzer, interview with author, March 8, 2019.

103 *Didn't think she (or any woman) had what it took:* Switzer, "The Real Story."

103 *Briefly considered dropping out:* Switzer, "The Real Story."

103 *Bodychecked:* Kathrine Switzer, *Marathon Woman: Running the Race to Revolutionize Women's Sports* (Cambridge, MA: Da Capo Press, 2009), 92.

103 *Four miles into the race:* Switzer, "The Real Story."

103 *Fear and humiliation:* Switzer, *Marathon Woman*, 93.

103 *Bloodied blisters:* Switzer, *Marathon Woman*, 108.

103 *"I'm in favor":* Myron Cope, "Angry Overseer of the Marathon," *Sports Illustrated*, April 22, 1968, 27.

104 *"Don't want to be a cheerleader":* Switzer, *Marathon Woman*, 8–9.

104 *"The mile a day":* Switzer, interview with author.

104 *"I am hurt to think":* Bob Sales, "Has Marathon Become Battle of Sexes?," *Boston Globe*, April 20, 1967, 52.

104 *"I would spank her":* Switzer, *Marathon Woman*, 118.

104 *Kicked out of the Amateur Athletic Union:* Switzer, *Marathon Woman*, 116–17.

105 *Marathon times:* Kathrine Switzer, "Accomplishments," accessed October 23, 2019, https://kathrineswitzer.com/accomplishments/.

105 *Jasmin Paris wins Spine Race:* Sean Ingle, "Jasmin Paris Becomes First Woman to Win 268-Mile Montane Spine Race," January 17, 2019, https://www.theguardian.com/sport/2019/jan/17/jasmin-paris-first-woman-win-gruelling-286-mile-montane-spine-race-ultrarunning.

105 *Spine Race gear:* Cassidy Randall, "Jasmin Paris on Her Record-Setting Win of Britain's Montane Spine Race," *Co-op Journal*, January 18, 2019, https://www.rei.com/blog/news/jasmin-paris-on-her-record-setting-win-of-britains-montane-spine-race.

105 *Winning time:* Derek Call, "Watch: Jasmin Paris Wins 268-Mile Race by More Than 15 Hours," RunnersWorld.com, January 27, 2019, https://www.runnersworld.com/news/a26038677/jasmin-paris-wins-268-mile-race-by-more-than-15-hours/.

105 *"A hobby":* Jasmin Paris, interview with author, May 1, 2019.

106 *Avoiding mastitis:* Paris, interview with author.

106 *"Any extra thing":* Paris, interview with author.

106 *Women are more accurate:* Anya Alvarez, "Men Are Stronger Than Women. But That Doesn't Make Them Better Athletes," *Guardian*, June 6, 2017, https://www.theguardian.com/sport/2017/jun/06/male-female-athlete-comparison-golf.

106 *"On the cusp":* Switzer, interview with author.

107 *"I don't know what that means":* Switzer, interview with author.

107 *Pedestrianism and competing activities:* Matthew Algeo, "The Insane 6-Day, 500-Mile Race That Riveted America," *Mental Floss*, March/April 2015, https://mentalfloss.atavist.com/the-insane-6-day-500-mile-race.

108 *Muscular Christianity:* Brett and Kate McKay, "When Christianity Was Muscular," ArtofManliness.com, accessed October 23, 2019, https://www.artofmanliness.com/articles/when-christianity-was-muscular/.

108 *Martin Luther:* McKay, "When Christianity Was Muscular."

108 *"The emerging crop":* McKay, "When Christianity Was Muscular."

109 *Boston YWCA:* "History," YWCA.org, accessed October 23, 2019, https://www.ywca.org/about/history/.

109 *"For muscle and manhood":* "Home Truths," *Revolution*, January 15, 1868, 17, https://archive.org/details/revolution-1868-01-15.

109 *"Grow up weaklings":* Maria Longworth Storer, *In Memoriam: Bellamy Storer; with personal remembrances of President McKinley, President Roosevelt and John Ireland, Archbishop of St. Paul* (Boston: Merrymount Press, 1923), 22.

112 *Gender polarization:* Sandra Lipsitz Bem, *The Lenses of Gender: Transforming the Debate on Sexual Inequality* (New Haven, CT: Yale University Press, 1993), 2.

112 *99.8 percent of their genes:* Lise Eliot, *Pink Brain, Blue Brain: How Small Differences Grow into Troublesome Gaps—and What We Can Do About It* (Oxford: Oneworld, 2012), 8.

112 *"Basic behavioral differences":* Robin McKie, "Male and Female Ability Differences Down to Socialisation, Not Genetics," August 14, 2010, https://www.theguardian.com/world/2010/aug/15/girls-boys-think-same-way.

112 *Crash-test dummies:* Caroline Criado-Perez, "The Deadly Truth About a

World Built for Men – from Stab Vests to Car Crashes," *Guardian,* February 23, 2019, https://www.theguardian.com/lifeandstyle/2019/feb/23/truth-world-built-for-men-car-crashes.

113 *Unspoken agreement:* Switzer, interview with author.

113 *Gender-neutral names:* Associated Press, "Why Gender-Neutral Baby Names Are on the Rise," *New York Post,* March 21, 2018, https://nypost.com/2018/03/21/why-gender-neutral-baby-names-are-on-the-rise/.

113 *Roughly 1 in 1,666:* "How Common Is Intersex?," Intersex Society of North America, accessed October 23, 2019, https://isna.org/faq/frequency/.

114 *Gender-reveal parties:* Diane Stopyra, "Dear Parents-to-Be: Stop Celebrating Your Baby's Gender," *Marie Claire,* July 5, 2017, https://www.marieclaire.com/culture/a28016/gender-reveal-parties/.

114 *"Kids rise or fall":* Eliot, *Pink Brain, Blue Brain,* 15.

114 *Activities associated with the opposite sex:* Kim Parker, Juliana Menasce Horowitz, and Renee Stepler, "On Gender Differences, No Consensus on Nature vs. Nurture," December 5, 2017, https://www.pewsocialtrends.org/2017/12/05/on-gender-differences-no-consensus-on-nature-vs-nurture/.

114 *"Girls who ventured":* Switzer, interview with author.

115 *"About 25 percent as good":* Jesse Greenspan, "When Billie Beat Bobby," History.com, last updated August 22, 2018, https://www.history.com/news/billie-jean-king-wins-the-battle-of-the-sexes-40-years-ago.

115 *"The bedroom and the kitchen":* Earl Gustkey, "Battle of the Sexes on a Tennis Court," *Los Angeles Times,* August 24, 2005, https://www.latimes.com/archives/la-xpm-2005-aug-24-et-book24-story.html.

115 *5-2 favorite:* Associated Press, "King vs. Riggs," *Morning News,* September 20, 1973, 35.

115 *"Jock mentality":* Nancy Woodhull, "King-Riggs Coverage: It's Awful," *Detroit Free Press,* September 9, 1973, D1.

115 *"Crack up":* Associated Press, "King vs. Riggs."

115 *"I said a lot of things":* David Pincus, "9/20/1973—The Battle of the Sexes," SBNation.com, September 20, 2010, https://www.sbnation.com/2010/9/20/1074055/9-20-1973-the-battle-of-the-sexes.

116 *Ann Trason:* Dowling, *The Frailty Myth,* 172.

116 *"I still hear people":* Barclay Stockett, interview with author, May 17, 2019.

116 *"The sooner little boys":* Leslie A. Heaphy and Mel Anthony May, editors, *Encyclopedia of Women and Baseball* (Jefferson, NC: McFarland & Company, 2006), 174.

117 *"It's a short leap":* Nelson, *The Stronger Women Get,* 7.

CHAPTER 8

119 *Calydonian Boar hunt:* Shmoop Editorial Team, "The Calydonian Boar Hunt Summary," Shmoop University, last modified November 11, 2008, https://www.shmoop.com/calydonian-boar-hunt/summary.html.

119 *Real . . . basketball game:* Sally Jenkins, "History of Women's Basketball, WNBA.com, July 3, 1997, https://www.wnba.com/news/history-of-womens-basketball/.

119 *1972 Boston Marathon:* Jerry Nason, "Women Officially Acknowledged in BAA Race," *Boston Globe*, April 17, 1972, http://archive.boston.com/marathon/history/1972.shtml.

119 *Janet Guthrie:* "Indy 500 Pioneer Janet Guthrie Savors the Day She Made History," *NPR*, May 17, 2018, https://www.npr.org/2018/05/27/613655708/indy-500-pioneer-janet-guthrie-savors-the-day-she-made-history.

120 *One in twenty-seven . . . to one in four:* Betsey Stevenson, "Beyond the Classroom: Using Title IX to Measure the Return to High School Sports," *The Review of Economics and Statistics* 92, no. 2 (May 2010): 284–301.

120 *Log tossing and marriage:* Miles Hutson, "Former Weightlifters Terry and Jan Todd Call Austin Their Home," *Daily Texan*, November 30, 2012, http://www.dailytexanonline.com/news/2012/11/30/former-weightlifters-terry-and-jan-todd-call-austin-their-home.

121 *Scotland's manhood stones: Stoneland*, directed by Todd Sansom, USA: Rogue Fitness, 2016, https://www.roguefitness.com/theindex/documentary/stoneland.

121 *Guinness World Record:* "Jan Todd," USAPowerlifting.com, accessed October 24, 2019, https://www.usapowerlifting.com/womens-hall-of-fame/jan-todd/.

121 *400 and 545.5 pounds:* USAPowerlifting.com, "Jan Todd."

121 *Terry told Jan:* Terry Todd, "A Legend in the Making," *Sports Illustrated,* November 5, 1979, 46.

121 *332.49 kilograms:* "The Dinnie Stones: The Ultimate Challenge," TheDinnieStones.com, accessed October 24, 2019, http://www.thedinniestones.com/.

121 *Named after Donald Dinnie:* Todd, "A Legend in the Making," 46–47.

122 *"Brutal-looking rocks":* Todd, "A Legend in the Making," 50.

122 *Whisky distributor:* Todd, "A Legend in the Making," 47.

122 *"We soon left":* Todd, "A Legend in the Making," 47.

123 *Attempting to lift:* Todd, "A Legend in the Making," 50.

123 *"For the whisky man":* Todd, "A Legend in the Making," 50.

123 *History of weightlifting:* "Weightlifting," Olympic.org, accessed October 24, 2019, https://www.olympic.org/weightlifting.

126 *"To get the weight":* Karyn Marshall, interview with author, May 15, 2019.

126 *"Fell in love":* Marshall, interview with author.

126 *Asked her coach:* Arthur Drechsler, "Karyn Marshall—USAW's First Overall Women's World Champion," TeamUSA.org, April 5, 2011, https://www.teamusa.org/usa-weightlifting/features/2011/april/05/karyn-marshall-usaw-s-first-overall-women-s-world-champion.

126 *By one vote:* Drechsler, "Karyn Marshall."

126 *Forty-five national records:* Lindsey Konkel, "First Women's Weightlifting Champ Reflects on Shattering Stereotypes," TEDxAsburyPark.com, August 15, 2016, https://tedxasburypark.com/08/2016/first-women-weightlifting-champ-shattering-stereotypes/.

126 *Sandwina's record and 300 pounds:* Drechsler, "Karyn Marshall."

127 *"I just felt this destiny":* Marshall, interview with author.

127 *"Not afraid of hard work":* Marshall, interview with author.

128 *"Not just about your physical strength":* Marshall, interview with author.

128 *Pudgy for reassurance:* Todd, "The Legacy of Pudgy Stockton," 7.

128 *Nude weigh-ins and jockstraps:* Sarah Pileggi, "The Pleasure of Being the World's Strongest Woman," *Sports Illustrated,* November 14, 1977, 64.

128 *Manspreading:* Olivia Petter, "Revealed: The Scientific Explanation Behind 'Manspreading,'" *Independent,* July 27, 2017, https://www.independent

.co.uk/life-style/manspreading-scientific-explanation-revealed-men-behaviour-public-transport-etiquette-a7862771.html.

129 *"An attribute of all humanity":* Dennis Breo and Susan Jack, "That's Not a Heavy Date but the 280-Lb. Husband of Jan Todd, the World's Strongest Woman," January 29, 1979, https://people.com/archive/thats-not-a-heavy-date-but-the-280-lb-husband-of-jan-todd-the-worlds-strongest-woman-vol-11-no-4/.

CHAPTER 9

131 *All Elaine Craig information:* Elaine Craig, interview with author, February 13, 2019.

132 *Bodybuilding's origins:* David Robson, "A History Lesson in Bodybuilding," Bodybuilding.com, July 16, 2019, https://www.bodybuilding.com/fun/drobson61.htm.

133 *Trip to Italy:* CandyGuy, "Eugen Sandow—Father of Bodybuilding," The HumanMarvels.com, December 20, 2007, https://www.thehumanmarvels.com/eugen-sandow-father-of-bodybuilding/.

133 *"Incalculable evils":* Jake Rossen, "15 Fitness Tips from 1800s Bodybuilder Eugen Sandow That Are Still Good Today," *Mental Floss,* December 23, 2016, http://mentalfloss.com/article/88665/15-fitness-tips-1800s-bodybuilder-eugen-sandow-are-still-good-today.

133 *"You might expect a documentary":* Gene Siskel, " 'Pumping Iron II' Develops Human Side of Bodybuilding," *Chicago Tribune,* May 31, 1985, https://www.chicagotribune.com/news/ct-xpm-1985-05-31-8502030911-story.html.

133 *Scenes in movie: Pumping Iron II: The Women,* directed by George Butler, USA: White Mountain Films, 1985.

134 *"When a woman came out":* Steve Wennerstrom, interview with author, February 15, 2019.

134 *Fred Howell:* Fred Howell, "Women's Bodybuilding: The State of the Art," unknown publication and date, 40–43, 52.

135 *Explaining his vision:* Dan Levin, "Here She Is, Miss, Well, What?," *Sports Illustrated,* March 17, 1980, 74–75.

135 *"Men don't monopolize strength":* Levin, "Here She Is," 74.

135 *"Challenge their physicality":* Wennerstrom, interview with author.

136 *"Judges sometimes look":* Levin, "Here She Is," 67.

136 *"I don't believe in all this muscle stuff":* Kate Santich, "Body by Doris," *Orlando Sentinel,* May 5, 1991, https://www.orlandosentinel.com/news/os-xpm-1991-05-05-9105041205-story.html.

136 *Photo with biceps flexed:* Jan Todd and Désirée Harguess, "Doris Barrilleaux and the Beginnings of Modern Women's Bodybuilding," *Iron Game History,* January 2012, 8–9.

136 *"Female physique contests should be discontinued":* Levin, "Here She Is," 73.

136 *IFBB published guidelines:* Susan Fry and Bill Dobbins, "Guidelines for Women's Bodybuilding Competition," International Federation of Bodybuilding and Fitness, November 1980.

137 *"With her squat chest":* Siskel, "Pumping Iron II."

138 *All Dana Linn Bailey quotes:* Dana Linn Bailey, interview with author, February 18, 2019.

CHAPTER 10

143 *Katrin Davidsdottir background:* Katrin Davidsdottir, interview with author, March 7, 2019.

145 *Symmetry suggests good genes:* Anthony C. Little, Benedict C. Jones, and Lisa M. DeBruine, "Facial Attractiveness: Evolutionary Based Research," *Philosophical Transactions of the Royal Society B: Biological Sciences* 366, no. 1571 (2011): 1638–59, https://dx.doi.org/10.1098%2Frstb.2010.0404.

145 *And youthfulness:* Olivia E. Linden, Jun Kit He, Clinton S. Morrison, Stephen R. Sullivan, and Helena O. B. Taylor, "The Relationship between Age and Facial Asymmetry," *Plastic and Reconstructive Surgery* 142, no. 5 (November 2018): 1145–1152, https://doi.org/10.1097/PRS.0000000000004831.

145 *Perfect symmetry to be creepy:* Emerson Rosenthal, "Photo Series Constructs Symmetrical Faces to Test Traditional Notions of Beauty," *Vice,* June 3, 2014, https://www.vice.com/en_us/article/ez5ne4/both-sides-of-explores-the-uncanny-imperfections-of-symmetry.

145 *Ancient Egyptian and Greek preferences:* "Women's Ideal Body Types Throughout History," BuzzFeed, June 2017, https://www.buzzfeed.com/watch/video/5088.

145 *Redheads and blondes:* Bettany Hughes, "Would You Be Beautiful in the Ancient World?," *BBC News Magazine*, January 10, 2015, https://www.bbc.com/news/magazine-30746985.

145 *1920s and 1980s:* "See How Much the 'Perfect' Female Body Has Changed in 100 Years (It's Crazy!)," *Greatist*, accessed October 25, 2019, https://greatist.com/grow/100-years-womens-body-image#1.

146 *Ironized Yeast Company ad:* Tamara Abraham, "'Add 5lb of Solid Flesh in a Week!' The Vintage Ads Promoting Weight Gain," *Daily Mail*, November 30, 2011, https://www.dailymail.co.uk/femail/article-2067821/Add-5lb-solid-flesh-week-The-vintage-ads-promoting-weight-GAIN.html.

146 *"To have a strong and muscular body":* Lewis, *Our Girls*, 69.

146 *"It is true":* Lewis, *Our Girls*, 70–71.

146 *"The people we're around":* Linda Lin, interview with author, October 19, 2018.

146 *"Women with muscles":* Daniel Kunitz, *Lift: Fitness Culture, from Naked Greeks and Acrobats to Jazzercise and Ninja Warriors* (New York: Harper Wave, 2016), 276.

148 *"I know people think":* Wright Thompson, "CrossFitter Katrin Davidsdottir Embodies the Legendary Icelandic Warrior," ESPN.com, September 6, 2019, https://www.espn.com/espn/story/_/id/27495747/crossfitter-katrin-davidsdottir-represents-iceland-history-strong-women-body-issue-2019.

148 *"Learned to love my muscles":* Simone Biles, "Simone Biles: How I Learned to Love My Muscles after Years of Covering Them Up," *Today*, January 9, 2018, https://www.today.com/series/love-your-body/olympian-simone-biles-why-she-loves-her-muscular-arms-t120860.

149 *Fifteen times more of it:* David J. Handelsman, Angelica L. Hirschberg, and Stéphane Bermon, "Circulating Testosterone as the Hormonal Basis of Sex Differences in Athletic Performance," *Endocrine Reviews* 39, no. 5 (October 2018): 803–29, https://doi.org/10.1210/er.2018-00020.

149 *Women can build muscle:* Greg Nuckols, "Strength Training for Women:

Setting the Record Straight," StrongerByScience.com, April 9, 2018, https://www.strongerbyscience.com/strength-training-women/.

149 *"For most of history":* Lin, interview with author.

149 *"Women are the enforcers":* J. C. Herz, *Learning to Breathe Fire: The Rise of CrossFit and the Primal Future of Fitness* (New York: Three Rivers Press, 2014), 235.

150 *2009 survey:* Leigh Peele, "Defining Bulky, Once and for All," LeighPeele.com, accessed October 25, 2019, https://www.leighpeele.com/bulky-muscles-and-training-females-the-definition.

150 *Background on Misty Copeland:* Misty Copeland with Charisse Jones, *Life in Motion: An Unlikely Ballerina* (New York: Touchstone Books, 2014).

151 *"Though I have tremendous support":* Jane Mulkerrins, "Misty Copeland: Meet the Ballerina Who Rewrote the Rules of Colour, Class and Curves," *Telegraph,* June 21, 2015, https://www.telegraph.co.uk/culture/theatre/dance/11675707/Misty-Copeland-ballerina-interview.html.

154 *"It's pretty crazy":* Misty Copeland, "Misty Copeland on Why She Loves Her 'Ripped' Back: 'I See My Strength as Beauty,'" *Today,* October 18, 2016, https://www.today.com/series/love-your-body/misty-copeland-why-she-loves-her-ripped-back-t103309.

154 *"I can't even watch":* Jaime Schultz, "Reading the Catsuit," *Journal of Sport & Social Issues* 29, no. 3 (August 2005): 346.

154 *"Hit the ball too hard":* Krystyna Rudzki, "Sabatini Lashes Boring Sister Act," *Independent,* June 24, 2002, https://www.independent.ie/sport/sabatini-lashes-boring-sister-act-26045710.html.

154 *Likened them to Amazons:* Nadra Nittle, "The Serena Williams Catsuit Ban Shows That Tennis Can't Get Past Its Elitist Roots," *Vox,* August 28, 2018, https://www.vox.com/2018/8/28/17791518/serena-williams-catsuit-ban-french-open-tennis-racist-sexist-country-club-sport.

154 *"I hate my muscles":* Schultz, "Reading the Catsuit."

154 *"The Williams brothers":* Christopher Clarey, "Russian Official Is Penalized for Williams Sisters Remark," *New York Times,* October 17, 2014, https://www.nytimes.com/2014/10/18/sports/tennis/wta-suspends-russian-official-for-comment-about-williams-sisters.html.

155 *"It's our decision":* Ben Rothenberg, "Tennis's Top Women Balance Body Image with Ambition," *New York Times*, July 10, 2015, https://www.nytimes.com/2015/07/11/sports/tennis/tenniss-top-women-balance-body-image-with-quest-for-success.html.

155 *"Now every girl":* Tina Fey, *Bossypants* (New York: Little, Brown and Company, 2011): 44–45, OverDrive.

155 *"My younger self":* Biles, "How I Learned to Love My Muscles."

CHAPTER 11

157 *"Confidence is where the page has turned":* Kunitz, *Lift*, 274.

157 *All Lei Wang information:* Lei Wang, interview with author, April 16, 2019.

161 *Ernst & Young found:* "Women Athletes Business Network," EY.com, accessed May 30, 2019, https://www.ey.com/br/pt/about-us/our-sponsorships-and-programs/women-athletes-global-leadership-network-perspectives-on-sport-and-teams.

161 *"Instead of just enjoying":* Macy, *Winning Ways*, 187.

161 *Attend college:* National Federation of State High School Associations, "The Case for High School Activities," NFHS.org, accessed October 25, 2019, https://www.nfhs.org/articles/the-case-for-high-school-activities/.

161 *Find a well-paying job:* Stevenson, "Beyond the Classroom."

161 *Work in male-dominated industries:* Rebecca Hinds, "The 1 Trait 94 Percent of C-Suite Women Share (and How to Get It)," *Inc.*, February 8, 2018, https://www.inc.com/rebecca-hinds/the-1-trait-94-percent-of-c-suite-women-share-and-how-to-get-it.html.

162 *Dianabol study:* Gideon Ariel and William Saville, "Anabolic Steroids: The Physiological Effects of Placebos," *Medicine and Science in Sports* 4, no. 2 (1972): 124–26.

162 *Powerlifters study:* Constantinos N. Maganaris, Dave Collins, and Martin Sharp, "Expectancy Effects and Strength Training: Do Steroids Make a Difference?," *Sport Psychologist* 14, no. 3 (2000): 272–78.

163 *"May just never happen":* "Fitness: Why Even Fit Women Can't Do Pull-

Ups," *Best Health*, accessed October 25, 2019, https://www.besthealthmag.ca/blog-post/fitness-why-even-fit-women-cant-do-pull-ups/.

163 *After three months:* Tara Parker-Pope, "Why Women Can't Do Pull-Ups," *New York Times Magazine*, October 28, 2012, https://well.blogs.nytimes.com/2012/10/25/why-women-cant-do-pull-ups/.

163 *"A more sinister effect":* Kyle Hill, "The Mechanics of the Pull-Up (and Why Women Can Absolutely Do Them)," ScientificAmerican.com, March 14, 2013, https://blogs.scientificamerican.com/guest-blog/the-mechanics-of-the-pull-up-and-why-women-can-absolutely-do-them/.

166 *All Liefia Ingalls quotes:* Liefia Ingalls, interview with author, March 21, 2019.

167 *Two days of competition:* Alissa Widman Neese, "Arnold's Strongwoman Contest Proves Powerful Women Can Pack a Crowd," *Columbus Dispatch*, March 4, 2017, https://www.dispatch.com/news/20170304/arnolds-strong woman-contest-proves-powerful-women-can-pack-crowd.

167 *Final two events:* FloElite video, "2017 Arnold Pro Strongwoman—Finals," commentary by Mike Gill, posted March 8, 2017, https://www.floelite.com/video/5759921-2017-arnold-pro-strongwoman-finals.

168 *Custom-made of solid bronze:* FloElite, "2017 Arnold Pro Strongwoman."

168 *Our brains will always tell us:* Brett and Kate McKay, "Dig Deep: You're Stronger Than You Think," ArtofManliness.com, last updated October 21, 2018, https://www.artofmanliness.com/articles/dig-deep-youre-stronger-than-you-think/.

169 *Hewlett-Packard internal report:* Katty Kay and Claire Shipman, "The Confidence Gap," *Atlantic*, May 2014, https://www.theatlantic.com/magazine/archive/2014/05/the-confidence-gap/359815/.

CHAPTER 12

171 *"Thrilled when we get crumbs":* Joshua Barajas, "Equal Pay for Equal Play. What the Sport of Tennis Got Right," *PBS NewsHour*, April 12, 2016, https://www.pbs.org/newshour/economy/equal-pay-for-equal-play-what-the-sport-of-tennis-got-right.

171 *Bonuses for teams:* Natasha Frost, "The US Women's Soccer Team

Is Suing over Gender Discrimination," *Quartz,* March 8, 2019, https://qz.com/1568831/the-us-womens-soccer-team-is-suing-for-equal-pay/.

171 *Sued U.S. Soccer:* Frost, "US Women's Soccer Team Is Suing."

172 *Controversy over goals:* Christianna Silva, "No, the USWNT Didn't Score 'Too Many' Goals or Celebrate 'Too Much,'" *MTV News,* June 12, 2019, http://www.mtv.com/news/3127072/uswnt-world-cup-win-13-0-thailand/.

172 *"Some sort of double standard":* Alex Morgan, press conference, July 5, 2019.

172 *"It's just been true":* Christen Press and Megan Rapinoe, "Next Step in Equal Pay Fight," interview by Savannah Guthrie, *Today,* August 15, 2019, https://www.nbcnews.com/news/sports/u-s-women-s-soccer-team-ready-take-fair-pay-n1042566.

173 *Heidi Stevens:* Heidi Stevens, "Column: Boys Are Wearing U.S. Women's National Team Jerseys and That Feels like Progress," *Chicago Tribune,* June 20, 2019, https://www.chicagotribune.com/columns/heidi-stevens/ct-heidi-stevens-thursday-boys-wearing-womens-soccer-jerseys-0620-20190620-7qgm7t2j2rgonkosjfjwm4digq-story.html.

173 *2 percent of airtime:* Cheryl Cooky, Michael A. Messner, and Michela Musto, "It's Dude Time!": A Quarter Century of Excluding Women's Sports in Televised News and Highlight Shows," *Communication and Sport* 3, vol. 3 (September 1, 2015): 266.

173 *Not even half a percent of sponsorship money:* Janet S. Fink, "Sponsorship for Women's Sports Presents Untapped Opportunity," *Sports Business Journal,* November 2, 2015, https://www.sportsbusinessdaily.com/Journal/Issues/2015/11/02/Opinion/Changing-the-Game-Janet-Fink.aspx.

174 *Allyson Felix . . . spoke out:* Allyson Felix, "Allyson Felix: My Own Nike Pregnancy Story," *New York Times,* May 22, 2019, https://www.nytimes.com/2019/05/22/opinion/allyson-felix-pregnancy-nike.html.

174 *Kara Goucher had her pay:* Alysia Montaño, "Nike Told Me to Dream Crazy, Until I Wanted a Baby," *New York Times,* May 12, 2019, https://www.nytimes.com/2019/05/12/opinion/nike-maternity-leave.html.

174 *Felix . . . with Athleta:* Morgan M. Evans, "Olympic Sprinter Allyson Felix Has a New Partnership That's Championing Female Athletes and Mothers," People.com, July 31, 2019, https://people.com/sports/allyson-felix/.

174 *Nike agreed to amend its contracts:* Chris Chavez, "Nike Removes Contract Reductions for Pregnant Athletes After Backlash," *Sports Illustrated,* August 16, 2019, https://www.si.com/olympics/2019/08/16/nike-contract-reduction-pregnancy-protection-athlete-maternity-leave.

174 *Fewer covers of* Sports Illustrated*:* Jonetta D. Weber and Robert M. Carini, "Where Are the Female Athletes in *Sports Illustrated*? A Content Analysis of Covers (2000–2011)," *International Review for the Sociology of Sport* 48, vol. 2 (2013): 196–203.

174 *"Strong and angry women":* Karyn Marshall, "Shattering Records and Glass Ceilings," filmed April 11, 2015 at TEDxNavesink: Accelerators, West Long Branch, NJ.

175 *Equality in CrossFit:* Mike Warkentin, "Why Men and Women Are Always Equal in CrossFit," *CrossFit Journal,* July 15, 2018, https://journal.crossfit.com/article/equality-warkentin.

175 *"I really appreciate it":* Stockett, interview with author.

178 *The Rock Instagram post:* Dwayne Johnson (@therock), "I'm Callin' It Now," Instagram video, January 2, 2019, https://www.instagram.com/p/BsKA08dh9E8/. (This post was edited for clarity.)

178 *2017 season:* Mark Podolski, "'American Ninja Warrior' Executive Producer Says Women a Boon for the Show," *News-Herald,* May 7, 2017, https://www.news-herald.com/sports/american-ninja-warrior-executive-producer-says-women-a-boon-for/article_437b787d-8cb5-50f8-93da-fa2fb0df9538.html.

179 *"I was so intimidated":* Tia-Clair Toomey, interview with author, March 1, 2019.

180 *Female powerlifter statistics:* Dave Tate, "Subject: The State of Powerlifting," EliteFTS.com, March 13, 2017, https://www.elitefts.com/coaching-logs/subject-the-state-of-powerlifting/.

180 *Stefi Cohen:* Jake Boly, "Stefi Cohen Squats a Massive 495 lb PR and Unofficial World Record," *BarBend,* March 2, 2019, https://barbend.com/stefi-cohen-squats-495-lbs/.

180 *Weightlifting female participation:* Will Cockrell, "Lift Off," *Red Bulletin,* July 1, 2018, https://www.redbull.com/us-en/theredbulletin/olympic-weightlifting-on-the-rise-with-women.

180 *Women's world records:* Dresdin Archibald, "But What Do They Mean? An Analysis of Weightlifting World Records," BreakingMuscle.com, accessed October 25, 2019, https://breakingmuscle.com/fitness/but-what-do-they-mean-an-analysis-of-weightlifting-world-records.

180 *"A personal adventure":* Kim Beckwith, interview with author, January 18, 2019.

181 *"Putting yourself out there":* Megan Rapinoe, "Dear Megan: A Letter to My 13-Year-Old Self," *Bleacher Report,* August 5, 2016, https://thelab.bleacherreport.com/dear-megan/.

AFTERWORD

184 *"Women are pigeonholed":* Wennerstrom, interview with author.

186 *"I was always interested":* Babe Didrikson Zaharias, *This Life I've Led: My Autobiography* (New York: A. S. Barnes, 1955), 104.

187 *Edie Edmundson:* Edie Edmundson, interviews with author, December 10, 2018, and February 7, 2019.

189 *"I've evolved over time":* Molly Galbraith, interview with author, May 13, 2019.